Chicken Soup

Soup for the

Woman's Soul

Stories to open the heart and rekindle the spirits of women

Jack Canfield

Mark Victor Hansen

Jennifer Read Hawthorne

Marci Shimoff

Vermilion
LONDON

We would like to acknowledge the following publishers and individuals for permission to reprint the following material. (Note: The stories that were penned anonymously, that are public domain, or that were written by Jennifer Read Hawthorne or Marci Shimoff are not included in this listing.)

(Continued on page 346)

10 9 8 7 6

Copyright © 1996 Jack Canfield, Mark Victor Hansen, Jennifer Read Hawthorne and Marci Shimoff

The right of Jack Canfield, Mark Victor Hansen, Jennifer Read Hawthorne and Marci Shimoff to be identified as the Authors of this work has been asserted by them in accordance with the Copyright, Designs and Patents Act, 1988.

All rights reserved. No part of this publication may be reproduced, stored in a retrieval system, or transmitted in any form or by any means, electronic, mechanical, photocopying, recording or otherwise, without the prior permission of the copyright owners.

Published by arrangement with Health Communications, Inc., 3201 S.W. 15th Street, Deerfield Beach, FL 33442-8190, USA.
This edition published in 1999 by Vermilion, an imprint of Ebury Press
Random House, 20 Vauxhall Bridge Road, London SW1V 2SA
www.randomhouse.co.uk

Random House UK Limited Reg. No. 954009

Papers used by Vermilion are natural, recyclable products made from wood grown in sustainable forests

Printed and bound in Great Britain by Mackays of Chatham plc, Kent

A CIP catalogue record for this book is available from the British Library

ISBN 0-09-182506-7

NOTE THE QUOTE!
"Courage is its most important virtue"
                    MAYA Angelou —

a phenomenal woman .....

This is for another

· · · · · Phenomenal Woman
— Mona Nashman-Smith

Pretty women wonder where my secret lies.
I'm not cute or built to suit a fashion model's size
But when I start to tell them,
They think I'm telling lies.
I say,
It's in the reach of my arms,
The span of my hips,
The stride of my step,
The curl of my lips.
I'm a woman
Phenomenally.
Phenomenal woman,
That's me.

I walk into a room
Just as cool as you please,
And to a man,
The fellows stand or
Fall down on their knees.
Then they swarm around me,
A hive of honey bees.
I say,
It's the fire in my eyes,
And the flash of my teeth,
The swing in my waist,
And the joy in my feet.
I'm a woman

Phenomenally.
Phenomenal woman,
That's me.

Men themselves have wondered
What they see in me.
They try so much
But they can't touch
My inner mystery.
When I try to show them
They say they can't see.
I say,
It's in the arch of my back,
The sun of my smile,
The ride of my breasts,
The grace of my style.
I'm a woman
Phenomenally.
Phenomenal woman,
That's me.

Now you understand
Just why my head's not bowed.
I don't shout or jump about
Or have to talk real loud.
When you see me passing
It ought to make you proud.
I say,
It's in the click of my heels,
The bend of my hair,
The palm of my hand,
The need for my care.
 'Cause I'm a woman
Phenomenally.
Phenomenal woman,
That's me.

Maya Angelou

Namasté dear Mona,
Sent with my warmost wishes and love,
Anna Scher

PEACE PEBBLES WORKSHOP OMAN 1—7 DECEMBER

Contents

3. OVERCOMING OBSTACLES

4. ON MARRIAGE

5. ON MOTHERHOOD

6. SPECIAL MOMENTS

7. LIVE YOUR DREAM

8. ON AGING

9. HIGHER WISDOM

10. ACROSS THE GENERATIONS

Acknowledgments

Chicken Soup for the Woman's Soul has taken more than a year to write, compile and edit. It has been a true labor of love for all of us. One of the greatest joys in creating this book has been working with people who gave this project not just their time and attention, but their hearts and souls as well. We would like to thank the following people for their dedication and contributions, without which this book could not have been created:

Our families, who have given us love and support throughout this project, and have been chicken soup for *our* souls!

Dan Hawthorne, for always believing in us and in the importance of this project. Dan, thank you for helping us to keep our perspective and take ourselves lightly. We deeply appreciate your love and wonderful sense of humor!

Rusty Hoffman, for his unconditional love, his extraordinary support, his huge heart and his Internet expertise. Rusty, thank you for continually reminding us to enjoy the moment. You are a true saint!

Maureen H. Read, for reading and giving us feedback on hundreds of stories, and for always being there and cheering us on. We love you!

Louise and Marcus Shimoff, for their eternal support and love. We thank you for your constant willingness to research anything we needed, and for being one of our best sources of stories. We love you!

Elinor Hall, who assisted in every aspect of this project, from managing the *Chicken Soup for the Woman's Soul* office to doing research and providing emotional support. No job was too big or too small, and we thank you for your love, your friendship and your bliss—we couldn't have done it without you!

Ron Hall, for his unbounded consciousness, vision and love.

Carol Kline, for her great skill in reading and researching hundreds of stories, and for interviewing several women and writing their important stories for inclusion in the book. Carol, we are so grateful for your constant love and friendship.

Joanna Cox, for countless hours spent typing the preliminary manuscript and for always being there for us with infinite patience. We loved your steadying influence, and we loved working with you!

Nancy Berg and Eileen Lawrence, for their first-class job of editing numerous stories for us. We deeply appreciate the way you were able to capture the essence of *Chicken Soup for the Soul* in the stories you worked on.

Dan Clark, for sharing many of his stories and for working long and late hours editing stories to enable us to meet our deadlines.

Suzanne Lawlor, for her research and her generous heart.

K. Bernard, Bobby Roth, Susan Shatkin, Emily Sledge and Mary Zeilbeck for their editing assistance.

Peter Vegso and Gary Seidler at Health Communications, Inc., for believing in this book from the moment it was proposed, and for getting it into the hands of millions of readers. Thank you, Peter and Gary!

Christine Belleris, Matthew Diener and Mark Colucci, our editors at Health Communications, Inc., for their generous efforts in bringing this book to its high state of excellence.

Kim Weiss and Arielle Ford for their brilliant public relations efforts.

Patty Aubery and Nancy Mitchell, coauthors of *Chicken Soup for the Surviving Soul,* who guided us through the process of creating this book and never wavered in their encouragement and inspiration. Patty, thank you for always being there with answers and understanding. Nancy, thank you for an outstanding job obtaining the permissions for the stories in this book.

Heather McNamara, for editing and preparing the final manuscript with such ease, talent and clarity. We deeply appreciate your patience and your valuable suggestions. You are a joy to work with!

Veronica Valenzuela and Julie Knapp, for helping in Jack's office to make sure everything ran smoothly.

Rosalie Miller (Auntie Ro), who nourished us with her food and her love in the final weeks of preparing the manuscript.

Barry Spilchuk, for sharing with us stories, cartoons, quotes—and cookies when needed. Barry, we greatly appreciate your encouragement and your sense of humor!

Mark Tucker, for telling his audiences across the country about this book. His efforts resulted in hundreds of stories being contributed.

Recie Mobley, Diane Montgomery and Jenny Bryson, for putting out a call for stories to the professional speakers in their companies.

Mavis Cordero and Women Inc., for supporting our project and inviting us to participate in their New York conference for women, "Uncommon Women on Common Ground."

Dan Fields, Elaine Glusac, Joann Landreth and Sheryl Vestal, for featuring *Chicken Soup for the Woman's Soul* in their publications.

Bonnie Bartlett and Elizabeth Caulder, for their enthusiastic support, and for spreading the word about our call for stories.

Aliza Sherman of Cybergirl Internet Media, for designing our Web page and getting us onto the Internet.

The following people, who completed the monumental task of reading the preliminary manuscript of the book, helped us make the final selections and made invaluable comments on how to improve the book: Patty Aubery, Kim Banks, Christine Belleris, Pamela Bice, Laura Chitty, Lane Cole, Debbie Davis, Linda Lowe DeGraaff, Pam Finger, Elinor Hall, Jean Hammond, Stephany Harward, Amy Hawthorne, Rachel Jorgensen, Kimberly Kirberger, Robin Kotok, Nancy Leahy, Jeanette Lisefski, Priscilla Lynch, Teresa Lynch, Barbara McLoughlin, Karen McLoughlin, Heather McNamara, Barbara McQuaide, Jackie Miller, Nancy Mitchell, Cindy Palajac, Debra Halperin Poneman, Maureen H. Read, Wendy Read, Carol Richter, Loren Rose, Marjorie E. Rose, Heather Sanders, Wendy Sheets, Louise and Marcus Shimoff, Carolyn Strickland, Paula Thomas, Debra Way and Kim Wiele. We truly thank you for your heroic contribution!

Craig Herndon, for his help in typing the manuscript and for managing all our data entry. Craig's work was instrumental in providing us with information from our manuscript readers to help us make our final selection of 101 stories.

Fairfield Printing, especially Stephany Harward and Deborah Roberts, for their enthusiastic support of the book and their willingness to put *Chicken Soup for the Woman's Soul* ahead of almost any printing project at any time.

Jim Rubis and the Fairfield Public Library, and Tony Kainauskas and 21st Century Bookstore, for their outstanding research assistance.

Rick and Irene Archer, for their artistic abilities and for their design of beautiful promotional materials.

Felicity and George Foster, for their talented design and color work.

Jerry Teplitz, for working with us on our cover design.

Terry Johnson, Bill Levacy and Blaine Watson, for their astute guidance on aspects of this project.

Georgia Noble, for opening her home to us in the final days of the project, and for sharing her light and love of beauty.

M., for the gifts of wisdom and knowledge.

The following people, who contributed through their emotional support and encouragement throughout the project: Amsheva Miller, Robert Kenyon, Lynn Robertson, Loren and Cliff Rose, Janet Jenkins, David and Sofia Deida and our support groups.

Many of the contributors to previous *Chicken Soup for the Soul* books, for their love of this project and their continued willingness to share their stories.

We also wish to acknowledge the hundreds of people who sent us stories, poems and quotes for possible inclusion in *Chicken Soup for the Woman's Soul.* While we were not able to use everything that was sent in, we were deeply touched by your heartfelt intention to share yourselves and your stories with us and our readers. Thank you!

Because of the enormity of this project, we may have left out the names of some people who helped us along the way. If so, we are sorry—please know that we really do appreciate all of you.

We are truly grateful for the many hands and hearts that made this book possible. We love you all!

With love we dedicate this book to
the 2.9 billion phenomenal women of the world.
May these stories touch your hearts
and inspire your souls.

We also dedicate this book to our parents,
Ellen Taylor and Fred Angelis, Una and Paul Hansen,
Maureen and Brooks Read, and Louise and
Marcus Shimoff, for the extraordinary gifts of
love and life you have given us.

Introduction

This book has been a gift to us. From the moment it was conceived, we have felt the love, joy and indomitable spirit of women every step of the way. Our hope is that this book will be a gift to you as well.

For many years the four of us have been speaking to audiences—often women's audiences—about living our lives more fully and joyfully. We've been inspired, even overwhelmed, by how eager women are to share their hearts, their stories and their lessons. It is from this inspiration that *Chicken Soup for the Woman's Soul* was born.

We experienced miracles every day in the creation of this book! We felt as if an invisible hand was guiding us along the way.

For example, we searched for more than a year for Phyllis Volkens, the author of "A Goodnight Kiss," to get her permission to use her story. We finally located a distant cousin, who told us that Phyllis and her husband had moved to Iowa, where they were living only miles from Jennifer and Marci! More remarkable, however, was the response of Phyllis's husband, Stanley, when we called. He told us how happy he was we had found them. They had been *Chicken Soup for the Soul* fans for years, but Phyllis had only about one week to live. He couldn't wait to tell her that she would be part of our book; he later told us how much it meant to her. She died two days later.

Women who sent us their stories told us repeatedly how grateful they were for the opportunity to write them down. They said that even if their stories were not included in our book, they were happy just to have expressed them. In doing so, they felt cleansed and renewed.

Because of this book we, too, are changed people. We see more clearly what's really important in life. We appreciate more deeply the human experience. And we live more fully in the moment.

Women bring such beautiful gifts to the world through their openness, compassion and wisdom. Our deepest desire is that each time you read these stories, you will come away with a greater appreciation for yourselves and for each other—as we all did.

As one of the women who wrote to us, Mary Michalica, so beautifully said:

> All women go through periods in their lives when numerous demands are placed on them—family, work, spouse, ex-spouse, children, stepchildren, parents.
>
> It is important, indeed necessary, to step back and re-evaluate one's priorities, to reflect on one's mission in life. For it is only in nurturing one's soul that one can nurture, take care of another. Sometimes, one must say, "Stop! Listen to me. I have a story to tell."

So from our hearts to yours, we offer you *Chicken Soup for the Woman's Soul.* May you experience the miracles of love and inspiration when you read this book. May it touch your heart and move your spirit.

Jack Canfield, Mark Victor Hansen,
Jennifer Read Hawthorne and Marci Shimoff

1

ON LOVE

The best and most beautiful things in the world cannot be seen or even touched. They must be felt with the heart.

Helen Keller

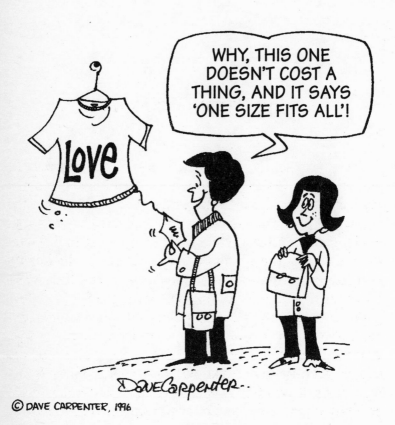

© DAVE CARPENTER, 1996

Reprinted with permission from Dave Carpenter.

The White Gardenia

Every year on my birthday, from the time I turned 12, one white gardenia was delivered anonymously to me at my house. There was never a card or note, and calls to the florist were in vain because the purchase was always made in cash. After a while, I stopped trying to discover the identity of the sender. I just delighted in the beauty and heady perfume of that one magical, perfect white flower nestled in folds of soft pink tissue paper.

But I never stopped imagining who the sender might be. Some of my happiest moments were spent in day-dreams about someone wonderful and exciting, but too shy or eccentric to make known his or her identity. In my teen years, it was fun to speculate that the sender might be a boy I had a crush on, or even someone I didn't know who had noticed me.

My mother often contributed to my speculations. She'd ask me if there was someone for whom I had done a special kindness, who might be showing appreciation anonymously. She reminded me of the times when I'd been riding my bike and our neighbor drove up with her car full of groceries and children. I always helped her unload the car and made sure the children didn't run into the road. Or maybe the mystery sender was the old man across the street. I often retrieved his mail during the winter, so he wouldn't have to venture down his icy steps.

My mother did her best to foster my imagination about the gardenia. She wanted her children to be creative. She also wanted us to feel cherished and loved, not just by her, but by the world at large.

When I was 17, a boy broke my heart. The night he called for the last time, I cried myself to sleep. When I awoke in the morning, there was a message scribbled on my mirror in red lipstick: "Heartily know, when half-gods go, the gods arrive." I thought about that quotation from Emerson for a long time, and I left it where my mother had written it until my heart healed. When I finally went for the glass cleaner, my mother knew that everything was all right again.

But there were some hurts my mother couldn't heal. A month before my high school graduation, my father died suddenly of a heart attack. My feelings ranged from simple grief to abandonment, fear, distrust and overwhelming anger that my dad was missing some of the most important events in my life. I became completely uninterested in my upcoming graduation, the senior-class play and the prom—events that I had worked on and looked forward to. I even considered staying home to attend college instead of going away as I had planned because it felt safer.

My mother, in the midst of her own grief, wouldn't hear of me missing out on any of these things. The day before my father died, she and I had gone shopping for a prom dress and had found a spectacular one—yards and yards of dotted Swiss in red, white and blue. Wearing it made me feel like Scarlett O'Hara. But it was the wrong size, and when my father died the next day, I forgot all about the dress.

My mother didn't. The day before the prom, I found that dress waiting for me—in the right size. It was draped majestically over the living room sofa, presented to me artistically and lovingly. I may not have cared about having a new dress, but my mother did.

She cared how we children felt about ourselves. She imbued us with a sense of the magic in the world, and she gave us the ability to see beauty even in the face of adversity.

In truth, my mother wanted her children to see themselves much like the gardenia—lovely, strong, perfect, with an aura of magic and perhaps a bit of mystery.

My mother died when I was 22, only 10 days after I was married. That was the year the gardenias stopped coming.

Marsha Arons

Words from the Heart

The bitterest tears shed over graves are for words left unsaid and deeds left undone.

Harriet Beecher Stowe

Most people need to hear those "three little words." Once in a while, they hear them just in time.

I met Connie the day she was admitted to the hospice ward, where I worked as a volunteer. Her husband, Bill, stood nervously nearby as she was transferred from the gurney to the hospital bed. Although Connie was in the final stages of her fight against cancer, she was alert and cheerful. We got her settled in. I finished marking her name on all the hospital supplies she would be using, then asked if she needed anything.

"Oh yes," she said, "would you please show me how to use the TV? I enjoy the soaps so much and I don't want to get behind on what's happening." Connie was a romantic. She loved soap operas, romance novels and movies with a good love story. As we became acquainted, she confided how frustrating it was to be married 32 years to a man who often called her "a silly woman."

"Oh, I know Bill loves me," she said, "but he has never been one to say he loves me, or send cards to me." She sighed and looked out the window at the trees in the courtyard. "I'd give anything if he'd say 'I love you,' but it's just not in his nature."

Bill visited Connie every day. In the beginning, he sat next to the bed while she watched the soaps. Later, when she began sleeping more, he paced up and down the hallway outside her room. Soon, when she no longer watched television and had fewer waking moments, I began spending more of my volunteer time with Bill.

He talked about having worked as a carpenter and how he liked to go fishing. He and Connie had no children, but they'd been enjoying retirement by traveling, until Connie got sick. Bill could not express his feelings about the fact that his wife was dying.

One day, over coffee in the cafeteria, I got him on the subject of women and how we need romance in our lives; how we love to get sentimental cards and love letters.

"Do you tell Connie you love her?" I asked (knowing his answer), and he looked at me as if I was crazy.

"I don't have to," he said. "She *knows* I do!"

"I'm sure she knows," I said, reaching over and touching his hands—rough, carpenter's hands that were gripping the cup as if it were the only thing he had to hang onto—"but she needs to *hear* it, Bill. She needs to hear what she has meant to you all these years. Please think about it."

We walked back to Connie's room. Bill disappeared inside, and I left to visit another patient. Later, I saw Bill sitting by the bed. He was holding Connie's hand as she slept. The date was February 12.

Two days later I walked down the hospice ward at noon. There stood Bill, leaning up against the wall in the hallway, staring at the floor. I already knew from the head nurse that Connie had died at 11 A.M.

When Bill saw me, he allowed himself to come into my arms for a long hug. His face was wet with tears and he was trembling. Finally, he leaned back against the wall and took a deep breath.

"I have to say something," he said. "I have to say how good I feel about telling her." He stopped to blow his nose. "I thought a lot about what you said, and this morning I told her how much I loved her . . . and loved being married to her. You shoulda seen her smile!"

I went into the room to say my own good-bye to Connie. There, on the bedside table, was a large Valentine card from Bill. You know, the sentimental kind that says, "To my wonderful wife . . . I love you."

Bobbie Lippman

Mama's Soup Pot

There are too many treasures in life we take for granted, the worth of which we don't fully realize until they're pointed out to us in some unexpected way. So it was with Mama's soup pot.

I can still see it sitting on the stove in all its chipped white-and-blue-enameled glory, its contents bubbling, steam rising as if from an active volcano. When I entered the back porch, the aroma was not only mouthwatering but reassuring. Whether Mama was standing over the pot stirring with a long wooden spoon or not, I knew I was home.

There was no recipe for her minestrone soup. It was always a work in progress. It had been so since her girlhood in the Piemonte mountains of northern Italy, where she learned its secret from her nonna (grandma), who had inherited it from generations of nonnas.

For our large immigrant family, Mama's soup guaranteed we would never go hungry. It was a simmering symbol of security. Its recipe was created spontaneously from what was in the kitchen. And we could judge the state of our family economy by its contents. A thick brew with tomatoes, pasta, beans, carrots, celery, onion, corn and meat indicated things were going well with the Buscaglias. A watery soup denoted meager times. And never was food thrown out. That was a sin against God. Everything ended up in the minestrone pot.

Its preparation was sacred to Mama. To her, cooking was a celebration of God's providence. Each potato, each shred of chicken was placed in the pot with grateful thanks. I think of Mama whenever I read Proverbs: "She gets up while it is still dark; she provides food for her family... Her children arise, and call her blessed."

At one time, however, Mama's soup pot became a source of embarrassment to me, for I feared it would cost me a new friend I had made at school. Sol was a thin, dark-haired boy, and an unusual pal for me because his father was a doctor and they lived in the best part of town. Often Sol invited me to his home for dinner. The family had a cook in a white uniform who worked in a kitchen of gleaming chrome and shining utensils. The food was good, but I found it bland, lacking the heartiness of my home fare served from flame-blackened pots. Moreover, the atmosphere matched the food. Everything was so formal. Sol's mother and father were polite, but conversation around the table was stilted and subdued. And no one hugged! The closest I saw Sol get to his father was a handshake.

In our family, warm hugs were a constant—men, women, boys and girls—and if you didn't kiss your mother, she demanded: "Whatsa matter, you sick?"

But at that time in my life, all this was an embarrassment.

I had known Sol would like to eat dinner at our house, but that was the last thing I wanted. My family was so different. No other kids had such pots on their stoves, nor did they have a mama whose first action upon seeing you enter the house was to sit you down with a spoon and bowl.

"People in America don't do things like that," I tried to convince Mama.

"Well, I'm not people," was her proud retort. "I'm Rosina. Only crazy people don't want my minestrone."

Finally Sol pointedly asked if he could come to our house. I had to say yes. I knew nothing would make Mama happier. But I was in a state of anxiety. Eating with my family would turn Sol off completely, I believed.

"Mama, why can't we have some American food like hamburgers or fried chicken?"

She fixed me with a stony glare and I knew better than to ask again.

The day Sol came over I was a nervous wreck. Mama and the other nine family members welcomed him with embraces and slaps on the back.

Soon we were sitting at the heavy, deeply stained and ornately carved table that was Papa's pride and joy. It was covered with an ostentatious, bright oilcloth.

And sure enough, after Papa asked the blessing, we were instantly faced with bowls of soup.

"Eh, Sol," Mama asked, "you know what this is?"

"Soup?" Sol responded.

"No soup," Mama said emphatically. "It's *minestrone!*" She then launched into a long, animated explanation of the power of minestrone: how it cured headaches, colds, heartaches, indigestion, gout and liver ailments.

After feeling Sol's muscles, Mama convinced him that the soup would also make him strong, like the Italian-American hero Charles Atlas. I cringed, convinced that this would be the last time I would ever see my friend Sol. He would certainly never return to a home with such eccentric people, odd accents and strange food.

But to my amazement, Sol politely finished his bowl and then asked for two more. "I like it a lot," he said, slurping.

When we were saying our good-byes, Sol confided, "You sure have a great family. I wish my mom could cook that good." Then he added, "Boy, are you lucky!"

Lucky? I wondered, as he walked down the street waving and smiling.

Today I know how lucky I was. I know that the glow Sol experienced at our table was much more than the physical and spiritual warmth of Mama's minestrone. It was the unalloyed joy of a family table where the real feast was love.

Mama died a long time ago. Someone turned off the gas under the minestrone pot the day after Mama was buried, and a glorious era passed with the flame. But the godly love and assurance that bubbled amidst its savory ingredients still warms my heart today.

Sol and I continued our friendship through the years. I was the best man at his wedding. Not long ago I visited his house for dinner. He hugged all his children and they hugged me. Then his wife brought out steaming bowls of soup. It was chicken soup, thick with vegetables and chunks of meat.

"Hey, Leo," Sol asked, "do you know what this is?"

"Soup?" I responded smiling.

"Soup!" he huffed. "This is *chicken soup!* Cures colds, headaches, indigestion. Good for your liver!" Sol winked.

I felt I was home again.

Leo Buscaglia

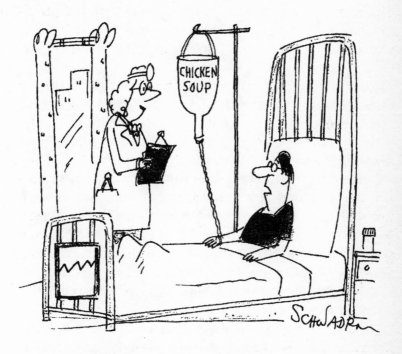

"Are you absolutely sure, Dr. Pleshke, that my mother's advice hasn't affected the treatment?"

Reprinted with permission from Harley Schwadron.

Just in Time

One night at 11:30, an older African-American woman was standing on the side of an Alabama highway trying to endure a lashing rain storm. Her car had broken down and she desperately needed a ride. Soaking wet, she decided to flag down the next car. A young white man stopped to help her—generally unheard of in the deep South during those conflict-filled 1960s. The man took her to safety, helped her get assistance and put her into a taxi cab. She seemed to be in a big hurry! She wrote down his address, thanked him and rode away.

Seven days went by and a knock came on the man's door. To his surprise, a giant combination console color TV and stereo record player were delivered to his home. A special note was attached. The note read:

Dear Mr. James:

Thank you so much for assisting me on the highway the other night. The rain drenched not only my clothes but my spirits. Then you came along. Because of you, I was able to make it to my dying husband's bedside just before he passed away. God bless you for helping me and unselfishly serving others.

Sincerely,
Mrs. Nat King Cole

Dan Clark

Gifts of the Heart

The love we give away is the only love we keep.

—Elbert Hubbard

In this hustle-bustle world we live in, it's so much easier to charge something on a credit card rather than give a gift of the heart.

And gifts of the heart are especially needed during the holidays.

A few years ago, I began to prepare my children for the fact that Christmas that year was going to be a small one. Their response was, "Yeah sure, Mom, we've heard that before!" I had lost my credibility because I had told them the same thing the previous year, while going through a divorce. But then I had gone out and charged every credit card to the max. I even found some creative financing techniques to pay for their stocking stuffers. This year was definitely going to be different, but they weren't buying it.

A week before Christmas, I asked myself, *What do I have that will make this Christmas special?* In all the houses we had lived in before the divorce, I had always made time to be the interior decorator. I had learned how to wallpaper, to lay wooden and ceramic tile, to sew curtains out of sheets and even more. But in this rental house there was little time for decorating and a lot less money. Plus, I was angry about this ugly place, with its red and orange carpets and turquoise and green walls. I refused to put money into it. Inside me, an inner voice of hurt pride shouted, *We're not going to be here that long!*

Nobody else seemed to mind about the house except my daughter Lisa, who had always tried to make her room her special place.

It was time to express my talents. I called my ex-husband and asked that he buy a specific bedspread for Lisa. Then I bought the sheets to match.

On Christmas Eve, I spent $15 on a gallon of paint. I also bought the prettiest stationery I'd ever seen. My goal was simple: I'd paint and sew and stay busy until Christmas morning, so I wouldn't have time to feel sorry for myself on such a special family holiday.

That night, I gave each of the children three pieces of stationery with envelopes. At the top of each page were the words, "What I love about my sister Mia," "What I love about my brother Kris," "What I love about my sister Lisa" and "What I love about my brother Erik." The kids were 16, 14, 10 and 8, and it took some convincing on my part to assure them that they could find just one thing they liked about each other. As they wrote in privacy, I went to my bedroom and wrapped their few store-bought gifts.

When I returned to the kitchen, the children had finished their letters to one another. Each name was written on the outside of the envelope. We exchanged hugs and goodnight kisses and they hurried off to bed. Lisa was given special permission to sleep in my bed, with the promise not to peek until Christmas morning.

I got started. In the wee hours of Christmas morn, I finished the curtains, painted the walls and stepped back to admire my masterpiece. Wait—why not put rainbows and clouds on the walls to match the sheets? So out came my makeup brushes and sponges, and at 5 A.M. I was finished. Too exhausted to think about being a poor "broken home," as statistics said, I went to my room and found Lisa spread-eagled in my bed. I decided I couldn't sleep with arms and legs all over me, so I gently lifted her up and tiptoed her into her room. As I laid her head on the pillow, she said, "Mommy, is it morning yet?"

"No sweetie, keep your eyes closed until Santa comes."

I awoke that morning with a bright whisper in my ear. "Wow, Mommy, it's beautiful!"

Later, we all got up and sat around the tree and opened the few wrapped presents. Afterward the children were given their three envelopes. We read the words with teary eyes and red noses. Then we got to "the baby of the family's" notes. Erik, at 8, wasn't expecting to hear anything nice. His brother had written: "What I love about my brother Erik is that he's not afraid of anything." Mia had written, "What I love about my brother Erik is he can talk to anybody!" Lisa had written, "What I love about my brother Erik is he can climb trees higher than anyone!"

I felt a gentle tug at my sleeve, then a small hand cupped around my ear and Eric whispered, "Gee, Mom, I didn't even know they liked me!"

In the worst of times, creativity and resourcefulness had given us the best of times. I'm now back on my feet financially, and we've had many "big" Christmases with lots of presents under the tree . . . but when asked which Christmas is our favorite, we all remember that one.

Sheryl Nicholson

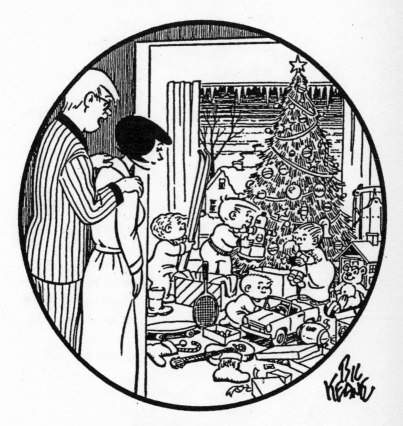

They won't know it till they're grown,
but their BEST gifts are the memories
they're making.

Reprinted with special permission of King Features Syndicate.

The Other Woman

After 21 years of marriage, I've discovered a new way of keeping the spark of love and intimacy alive in my relationship with my wife:

I've recently started dating another woman.

It was my wife's idea, actually. "You know you love her," she said one day, taking me by surprise. "Life is too short. You need to spend time with the people you love."

"But I love *you*," I protested.

"I know. But you also love her. You probably won't believe me, but I think that if the two of you spend more time together, it will bring the two of us closer."

As usual, Peggy was right.

The other woman that my wife was encouraging me to date was my mother.

My mom is a 71-year-old widow who has lived alone since my father died 19 years ago. Right after his death, I moved 2,500 miles away to California, where I started my own family and career. When I moved back near my hometown five years ago, I promised myself I would spend more time with her. But somehow with the demands of my job and three kids, I never got around to seeing her much beyond family get-togethers and holidays.

She was surprised and suspicious when I called and suggested the two of us go out to dinner and a movie. "What's wrong? Are you moving my grandchildren away?" she asked. My mother is the type of woman who thinks anything out of the ordinary—a late-night phone call or a surprise dinner invitation from her eldest son—signals bad news.

"I thought it would be nice to spend some time with you," I said. "Just the two of us."

She considered that statement for a moment.

"I'd like that," she said. "I'd like that a lot."

I found myself nervous as I drove to her house Friday after work. I had the pre-date jitters—and all I was doing was going out with my mother, for Pete's sake!

What would we talk about? What if she didn't like the restaurant I chose? Or the movie?

What if she didn't like either?

When I pulled into her driveway, I realized how excited she, too, was about our date. She was waiting by the door with her coat on. Her hair was curled. She was smiling. "I told my lady friends that I was going out with my son, and they were all impressed," she said as she got into my car. "They can't wait until tomorrow to hear about our evening."

We didn't go anywhere fancy, just a neighborhood place where we could talk. When we got there my mother clutched my arm—half out of affection and half to help her negotiate the steps into the dining room.

Once we were seated, I had to read the menu for both of us. Her eyes only see large shapes and shadows. Halfway through listing the entrées, I glanced up. Mom was sitting across the table, just looking at me. A wistful smile traced her lips.

"I used to be the menu reader when you were little," she said.

I understood instantly what she was saying. From care-giver to cared-for, from cared-for to caregiver; our rela-tionship had come full circle.

"Then it's time for you to relax and let me return the favor," I said.

We had a nice talk over dinner. Nothing earth-shattering, just catching up with each other's lives. We talked so much that we missed the movie. "I'll go out with you again, but only if you let me buy dinner next time," my mother said as I dropped her off. I agreed.

"How was your date?" my wife wanted to know when I got home that night.

"Nice . . . nicer than I thought it would be," I said.

She smiled her told-you-so smile.

Since that night I've been dating Mom regularly. We don't go out every week, but we try to see each other at least a couple of times a month. We always have dinner, and sometimes we take in a movie, too. Mostly, though, we just talk. I tell her about my daily trials at work. I brag about the kids and my wife. She fills me in on the family gossip I can never seem to keep up on.

She also tells me about her past. Now I know what it was like for my Mom to work in a factory during World War II. I know about how she met my father there, and how they nurtured a trolley-car courtship through those difficult times. As I've listened to these stories, I've come to realize how important they are to me. They are my his-tory. I can't get enough of them.

But we don't just talk about the past. We also talk about the future. Because of health problems, my mother wor-ries about the days ahead. "I have so much living to do," she told me one night. "I need to be there while my grand-children grow up. I don't want to miss *any* of it."

Like a lot of my baby-boomer friends, I tend to rush around, filling my At-A-Glance calendar to the brim as I struggle to fit a career, family and relationships into my life. I often complain about how quickly time flies. Spending time with my mom has taught me the importance of slowing down. I finally understand the meaning of a term I've heard a million times: quality time.

Peggy was right. Dating another woman *has* helped my marriage. It has made me a better husband and father, and hopefully, a better son.

Thanks, Mom. I love you.

David Farrell

Ramona's Touch

It was only a few weeks after my surgery, and I went to Dr. Belt's office for a checkup. It was just after my first chemotherapy treatment.

My scar was still very tender. My arm was numb underneath. This whole set of unique and weird sensations was like having a new roommate to share the two-bedroom apartment formerly known as my breasts—now lovingly known as "the breast and the chest."

As usual, I was taken to an examination room to have my blood drawn, again—a terrifying process for me, since I'm so frightened of needles.

I lay down on the examining table. I'd worn a big plaid flannel shirt and a camisole underneath. It was a carefully thought out costume that I hoped others would regard as a casual wardrobe choice. The plaid camouflaged my new chest, the camisole protected it and the buttons on the shirt made for easy medical access.

Ramona entered the room. Her warm sparkling smile was familiar, and stood out in contrast to my fears. I'd first seen her in the office a few weeks earlier. She wasn't my nurse on that day, but I remember her because she was laughing. She laughed in deep, round and rich tones. I remember wondering what could be so funny behind that medical door. What could she possibly find to laugh about at a time like this? So I decided she wasn't serious enough about the whole thing and that I would try to find a nurse who was. But I was wrong.

This day was different. Ramona had taken my blood before. She knew about my fear of needles, and she kindly hid the paraphernalia under a magazine with a bright blue picture of a kitchen being remodeled. As we opened the blouse and dropped the camisole, the catheter on my breast was exposed and the fresh scar on my chest could be seen.

She said, "How is your scar healing?"

I said, "I think pretty well. I wash around it gently each day." The memory of the shower water hitting my numb chest flashed across my face.

She gently reached over and ran her hand across the scar, examining the smoothness of the healing skin and looking for any irregularities. I began to cry gently and quietly. She brought her warm eyes to mine and said, "You haven't touched it yet, have you?" And I said, "No."

So this wonderful, warm woman laid the palm of her golden brown hand on my pale chest and she gently held it there. For a long time. I continued to cry quietly. In soft tones she said, "This is part of your body. This is you. It's okay to touch it." But I couldn't. So she touched it for me. The scar. The healing wound. And beneath it, she touched my heart.

Then Ramona said, "I'll hold your hand while you touch it." So she placed her hand next to mine, and we both were quiet. That was the gift that Ramona gave me.

That night as I lay down to sleep, I gently placed my hand on my chest and I left it there until I dozed off. I knew I wasn't alone. We were all in bed together, metaphorically speaking, my breast, my chest, Ramona's gift and me.

Betty Aboussie Ellis

"Are You God?"

One cold evening during the holiday season, a little boy about six or seven was standing out in front of a store window. The little child had no shoes and his clothes were mere rags. A young woman passing by saw the little boy and could read the longing in his pale blue eyes. She took the child by the hand and led him into the store. There she bought him some new shoes and a complete suit of warm clothing.

They came back outside into the street and the woman said to the child, "Now you can go home and have a very happy holiday."

The little boy looked up at her and asked, "Are you God, Ma'am?"

She smiled down at him and replied, "No son, I'm just one of His children."

The little boy then said, "I knew you had to be some relation."

Dan Clark

The Electric Candlesticks

Once a month on a Friday morning, I take a turn at the local hospital delivering Sabbath candlesticks to the Jewish female patients registered there. Lighting candles is the traditional way that Jewish women welcome the Sabbath, but hospital regulations don't allow patients to light real candles. So we offer the next best thing—electric candlesticks that plug in and are turned on at the start of the Jewish Sabbath on Friday at sundown. The Sabbath is over Saturday night. Sunday morning, I retrieve the candlesticks and store them away until the following Friday, when another volunteer comes to distribute them to that week's group of patients. Sometimes I see the same patients from the previous week.

One Friday morning, as I was making my rounds, I encountered a woman who was very old—perhaps 90. She had short snow-white hair that looked soft and fluffy, like cotton. Her skin was yellow and wrinkled, as if her bones had suddenly shrunk and left the skin around them with nothing to support it and nowhere to go; now it just hung in soft folds on her arms and face. She looked small there in the bed with the blanket pulled up under her arms. Her hands, resting on top of the cover, were gnarled and worn, the hands of experience. But her eyes were clear and blue, and her voice was surprisingly strong as she greeted me. From the list that the hospital had given me, I knew her name was Sarah Cohen.

She told me that she had been expecting me, that she never missed lighting candles at home and that I should just plug them in by the side of the bed where she could reach them. It was obvious that she was familiar with the routine.

I did as she asked and wished her a good Sabbath. As I turned to leave, she said, "I hope my grandchildren get here in time to say good-bye to me."

I think my face must have registered my shock at her matter-of-fact statement that she knew she was dying, but I touched her hand and said that I hoped so, too.

As I left the room, I almost collided with a young woman who looked to be about twenty or so. She wore a long skirt, peasant-style, and her hair was covered. I heard Mrs. Cohen say, "Malka! I'm glad you could get here. Where is David?"

I had to continue on my rounds, but a part of me could not help wondering if David would get there in time, too. It's hard for me to just deliver the candlesticks and leave, knowing that some of these patients are very sick, that some will probably die, and that they are someone's loved one. I suppose, in a way, each of these ladies reminds me of my mother when she was in the hospital, dying. I suppose that's why I volunteer.

All during the Sabbath, thoughts of Mrs. Cohen and her grandchildren kept intruding. On Sunday morning, I went back to the hospital to retrieve the candlesticks. As I approached Mrs. Cohen's room, I saw her grand-daughter sitting on the floor outside her door. She looked up as she heard my cart approach.

"Please," she asked, "could you leave the candlesticks for just a few more hours?"

I was surprised by her request, so she started to explain.

She told me that Mrs. Cohen had taught her and her brother, David, everything they knew about being religious. Their parents had divorced when they were very young and both parents had worked long hours. She and her brother spent most weekends with their grandmother.

"She made the Sabbath for us," said Malka. "She cooked and cleaned and baked and the whole house looked and smelled and was . . . special in a way I can't even express. Going there was like entering a different world. My brother and I found something there that did not exist anywhere else for us. I don't know how to make you understand what the Sabbath day meant for us—for all of us, Grandmother, David and me—but it was a respite from the rest of our lives. It was wonderful and it brought David and me back to our religion. David lives in Israel now. He couldn't get a flight out before today. He's supposed to be in around six, so if you could please leave the candlesticks until then, I'll gladly put them away after that."

I didn't understand what the candlesticks had to do with David's arrival. Malka explained. "Don't you see? For my grandmother, the Sabbath was our day for happiness. She wouldn't want to die on the Sabbath. If we could just make her believe that it's still the Sabbath, maybe she can hold on until David can get here. Just until he can tell her good-bye."

Nothing would have induced me to touch those candlesticks then, and I told Malka I would come back later. I couldn't say anything, so I just squeezed her hand.

There are some moments in time, some events, that can bond even total strangers. This was such a moment.

For the rest of the day, I went about my business but couldn't stop thinking about the drama unfolding at the hospital. Whatever strength that old lady in the hospital bed had left was being expended in just staying alive.

And it wasn't for herself that she was making the effort. She had already made it clear to me by her attitude that she didn't fear death. She had seemed to know and accept that it was her time, and was, in fact, ready to go.

For me, Sarah Cohen personified a type of strength I didn't know existed, and a type of love I didn't know could be so powerful. She was willing to concentrate her whole being on staying alive through the Sabbath. She didn't want her loved ones to associate the beauty and joy of the Sabbath with the sadness of her death. And perhaps she also wanted her grandchildren to have the sense of closure that comes from being able to say good-bye to the one person who most profoundly affected their lives.

When I returned to the hospital Sunday night, I was crying before I even reached the room. I looked inside. The bed was empty and the candlesticks had been turned off.

Then I heard a voice behind me say softly, "He made it."

I looked into Malka's dry-eyed face. "David arrived this afternoon. He's saying his prayers now. He was able to tell her good-bye and he also had good news—he and his wife are expecting a baby. If it's a girl, her name will be Sarah."

Somehow, I wasn't surprised.

I wrapped the electric cord around the base of the candlesticks. They were still warm.

Marsha Arons

More Than a Scholarship

*G*reat thoughts speak only to the thoughtful mind,
But great actions speak to all mankind.

Emily P. Bissell

You may have heard of Osceola McCarty. She's the 88-year-old woman in Mississippi who had worked for over 75 years as a washer woman. One day after she retired, she went to the bank and discovered, to her great surprise, that her meager monthly savings had grown to over $150,000. Then to *everyone's* great surprise, she turned around and donated $150,000—almost all of those savings—to the University of Southern Mississippi (USM) for a scholarship fund for African-American students with financial needs. She made national headlines.

What you have not heard is how Osceola's gift has affected my life. I am 19 years old and the first recipient of an Osceola McCarty Scholarship.

I was a dedicated student, and I had my heart set on going to USM. But I missed being eligible for a regular scholarship by one point on my entrance exams, and a scholarship was the only way I could attend.

One Sunday, I came across the story in the paper about Osceola McCarty and her generous gift. I showed my mother the article, and we both agreed it was a great thing to have done.

The next day I went to the financial aid office, and they told me there was still no money available for me, but if anything came up they'd call. A few days later, as I was running out the door to catch a ride with my mother to work, the phone rang. I stopped to pick it up, and while I heard my mother honking the horn for me to hurry up, they told me I had been chosen to receive the first Osceola McCarty Scholarship. I was ecstatic! I ran out as fast as I could to tell my mother. She had to call the office again herself to make sure it was true.

I first met Osceola at a press conference—meeting her was like finding family. Osceola never married or had children, so my family has since become her family. My grandma and she talk on the phone regularly and do errands together, and she joins us for family functions.

Once we got around to talking about ice cream. We found out Osceola hadn't had much experience with ice cream, so we all packed into the car and went to the Dairy Queen, where we ordered Osceola her first banana split! She has ice cream a lot now.

Osceola worked hard her whole life—from early in the morning to sunset—washing clothes by hand. I used to drive right by her house every day on my way to school. Of course, at the time I didn't know it was her house, but I did notice how well kept the lawn was and how everything was clean and neat. Recently I asked her why I never saw her once in all that time, and she answered, "I guess I was out in back, washing clothes."

Now that Osceola's retired, she sits most of the day and reads the Bible. That is, when she's not out getting awards! Every time I go visit, she has a new award. She's even gone to the White House. She is so happy and proud, though not at all conceited. We had to talk her into getting a VCR so she could tape the programs and see herself on TV—she just sits and smiles.

Osceola gave me much more than a scholarship. She taught me about the gift of giving. Now I know there are good people in the world who do good things. She worked her whole life and gave to others, and in turn she has inspired me to give back when I can. Eventually I plan to add to her scholarship fund.

I want to give Osceola the family she's always wanted, so I've adopted her as another grandma. She even calls me her granddaughter. And when I graduate from USM, she'll be sitting in the audience between my mother and my grandmother—right where she belongs.

Stephanie Bullock

It Couldn't Hurt

Random Acts of Kindness—huh!	It couldn't hurt.
I told my husband I love him.	It couldn't hurt.
I packed a note in my son's lunch box telling him how special he is.	It couldn't hurt.
I opened the door for a lady in a wheelchair at Walgreens.	It couldn't hurt.
I left a box of cookies for the mailman.	It couldn't hurt.
I let someone go in front of me in the grocery line.	It didn't hurt.
I called my brother to tell him I miss him.	He misses me too!
I sent the Mayor a note saying what a good job he is doing.	It couldn't hurt.
I took flowers to the nursing home.	It couldn't hurt.
I cooked some chicken soup for a friend who is sick.	It couldn't hurt.

I played Candy Land with my
daughter.

It was fun.

I thanked the person who bagged
my groceries.

He beamed.

I gave my assistant the day off
with pay.

It only hurt a little.

I played ball with my dog.

It felt good.

I invited a woman who doesn't
drive to lunch and to a movie.

I enjoyed myself.

I got a massage for me.

It felt marvelous.

Random Acts of Kindness—hmmm,
maybe I'll live this way all year.

It couldn't hurt.

Sandy Ezrine

A Goodnight Kiss

Every afternoon when I came on duty as the evening nurse, I would walk the halls of the nursing home, pausing at each door to chat and observe. Often, Kate and Chris would be sitting with their big scrapbooks in their laps and reminiscing over the photographs. Proudly, Kate showed me pictures of bygone years: Chris tall, blond and handsome; Kate pretty, dark-haired and laughing. Two young lovers smiling through the passing seasons. How lovely they looked, sitting together, the light from the window shining on their white heads, their time-wrinkled faces smiling at the memory of the years, caught and held forever in the scrapbooks.

How little the young know of loving, I'd think. How foolish to think they have a monopoly on such a precious commodity. The old know what loving truly means; the young can only guess.

As the staff members ate their evening meal, sometimes Kate and Chris, holding hands, would walk slowly by the dining room doors. Then the conversation would turn to a discussion of the couple's love and devotion, and what would happen when one of them died. We all knew Chris was the strong one, and Kate was dependent upon him.

How would Kate function if Chris were to die first? we often wondered.

Bedtime followed a ritual. When I brought the evening medication, Kate would be sitting in her chair, in nightgown and slippers, awaiting my arrival. Under Chris's and my watchful eyes, Kate would take her pill. Then very carefully Chris would help her from chair to bed and tuck the covers around her frail body.

Observing this act of love, I would think for the thousandth time, *Good heavens, why don't nursing homes have double beds for married couples?* All their lives they have slept together, but in a nursing home, they're expected to sleep in single beds. Overnight they're deprived of a comfort of a lifetime.

How very foolish such policies are, I would think as I watched Chris reach up and turn off the light above Kate's bed. Then tenderly he would bend, and they would kiss gently. Chris would pat her cheek, and both would smile. He would pull up the side rail on her bed, and only then would he turn and accept his own medication. As I walked into the hall, I could hear Chris say, "Good-night, Kate," and her returning voice, "Good-night, Chris," while the space of an entire room separated their two beds.

I had been off duty two days. When I returned, the first news I heard after walking through the nursing home doors was, "Chris died yesterday morning."

"How?"

"A massive heart attack. It happened quickly."

"How's Kate?"

"Bad."

I went into Kate's room. She sat in her chair, motionless, hands in her lap, staring. Taking her hands in mine, I said, "Kate, it's Phyllis."

Her eyes never shifted; she only stared. I placed my hand under her chin and slowly turned her head so she had to look at me.

"Kate, I just found out about Chris. I'm so sorry."

At the word "Chris," her eyes came back to life. She stared at me, puzzled, as though wondering how I had suddenly appeared. "Kate, it's me, Phyllis. I'm so sorry about Chris."

Recognition and remembrance flooded her face. Tears welled up and slid down her wrinkled cheeks. "Chris is gone," she whispered.

"I know," I said. "I know."

We pampered Kate for a while, letting her eat in her room, surrounding her with special attention. Then gradually the staff worked her back into the old schedule. Often, as I passed her room, I would observe Kate sitting in her chair, scrapbook on her lap, gazing sadly at pictures of Chris.

Bedtime was the worst part of her day. Although she had been granted her request to move from her bed to Chris's bed, and although the staff chatted and laughed with her as they tucked her in for the night, still Kate remained silent and sadly withdrawn. Passing her room an hour after she had been tucked in, I'd find her wide awake, staring at the ceiling.

The weeks passed, and the bedtime wasn't any better. Kate seemed so restless, so insecure. *Why?* I wondered. *Why this time of day more than the other hours?*

Then one night as I walked into her room, only to find the same wide-awake Kate, I said impulsively, "Kate, could it be you miss your good-night kiss?" Bending down, I kissed her wrinkled cheek.

It was as though I had opened the floodgates. Tears coursed down her face; her hands gripped mine. "Chris always kissed me good-night," she cried.

"I know," I whispered.

"I miss him so, all those years he kissed me good-night." She paused while I wiped the tears. "I just can't seem to go to sleep without his kiss."

She looked up at me, her eyes brimming with gratitude. "Oh, thank you for giving me a kiss."

A small smile turned up the corners of Kate's mouth. "You know," she said confidentially, "Chris used to sing me a song."

"He did?"

"Yes," her white head nodded, "and I lie here at night and think about it."

"How did it go?"

Kate smiled, held my hand and cleared her throat. Then her voice, small with age but still melodious, lifted softly in song:

So kiss me, my sweet, and so let us part.
And when I grow too old to dream,
that kiss will live in my heart.

Phyllis Volkens
Submitted by Jane Hanna

EDITORS' NOTE: Phyllis Volkens, the author of this story, died two days after we located her in an effort to obtain permission to use her story (see Introduction). Her husband, Stanley, told us how much it meant to Phyllis to be included in *Chicken Soup for the Woman's Soul.* We are honored to include "A Goodnight Kiss" in Phyllis's memory.

"When I Grow Too Old to Dream," lyrics by Oscar Hammerstein II, music by Sigmund Romberg. All rights reserved Robbins Music Corp.

Gifts

In my hands I hold a hardback copy of *Jules Verne's Classic Science Fiction*, torn airmail packaging scattered at my feet. The inscription: "To Matt, with love from Grandpa Loren, San Francisco." *Why is my 75-year-old father sending my 9-year-old son a 511-page book?* The inappropriateness of the gift irritates me—a gift hurriedly bought with too little care given. But perhaps it is unfair of me to expect my father to know what a boy of nine would like. Then I remember last spring, when we visited San Francisco. Dad sprinted after a cable car, grabbing Matt's hand and leaping aboard. Later he plucked a nickel off the street.

"Matt, look! When you put a coin on the track—the cable car almost cuts it in half!" I can still picture them standing there, heads bent in mutual admiration.

Less irritated, I stare out the window at Hondo, sleeping on the deck. He has been with us since he was eight weeks old. Gray hairs cover the muzzle of his glossy black head, and the lids beneath his brown eyes droop slightly. His huge Lab feet splay when he walks, more gray hairs grow from between his pads. I think of my father's beard and how I have watched the streaks of gray widen until gray is all there is.

Freckles rests next to Hondo, her border collie fur ruffling in the breeze. Much of her puppy freckling has faded. I think back to last summer.

Fourteen years represent a full life for a dog. Hondo's moon had begun to wane, growing weaker with the setting of each sun. The time for a second dog had come, but it was with guilt that we brought Freckles home to the ranch. When she scrambled out of the truck, puppy legs trembling, Hondo was a perfect gentleman. He sniffed and she cowered. She whined and he licked. Tails wagged, and a friendship was born.

Down at the barn, Freckles watched Hondo, a gracious teacher, sit patiently while we saddled the horses. She sat down as well. The cats rubbed up against Hondo's legs and Freckles learned not to chase cats. We rode out to check heifers, and Hondo trotted faithfully behind. Freckles learned that it was not all right to harass a cow or deer. Freckles grew lanky, and a new sprightliness came to Hondo's step. Years fell away. We began throwing sticks for him again, and he fetched until his panting jaws could no longer hold the stick. Freckles never learned to love the game, but she cheered him on anyway. He was given a brief reprieve, a second wind.

Then a hot summer day and too many miles traveled on dusty cow trails took their toll. Hondo collapsed in the corral. Soft coaxing and gentle stroking brought him around. Matt and Freckles looked on, watching him stagger to his feet and shake the dirt from his coat. Hondo drank deeply from the bucket by the house before climbing to the deck and taking up his post near the door. The next time we saddled the horses and rode out into the pasture, we locked him in the horse trailer. He peered through the wooden slats, his feelings hurt beyond comprehension.

"It's all right, old boy," I said, "we'll be back." But he had become deaf and did not hear me. After that we continued to take him with us on our rides. His moon will wane, no matter how protective we are.

I set the heavy volume of Jules Verne on the table and pick up the discarded packaging. Outside, a car drives by on the gravel road. Freckles hears the car and she stands, ears pricked forward. Hondo sleeps. Then Freckles barks, a quick and high-pitched sound—unlike the deep, chesty warning that has guarded our home for 14 years. It is not the noise of the car that finally awakens Hondo; the high-pitched bark penetrates his increasing deafness and he lifts his head to look about. He sees Freckles on duty, poised and ready. With a deep sigh of resignation, he lowers his head onto his paws and closes his eyes.

I want to go outside and take Hondo's gentle head in my hands, look into his brown eyes and speak softly, letting him feel with his heart those things he can no longer hear me say. I want him to cling to my world a little longer.

Instead, I pick up the book and reread the inscription. "To Matt, with love from Grandpa Loren." Suddenly the gift makes sense. Fourteen years separate Hondo and Freckles. Sixty-five years and a thousand miles separate my father from his grandson. Only a few more years of gift-giving stretch before him. He, too, counts the setting of each sun, watches the waning of his moon. Times does not allow him the luxury of sending only appropriate gifts. If in 10 years Matt opens this book, ready to dive 20,000 leagues beneath the sea, it will be his grandfather's words wishing him bon voyage.

Putting the heavy volume down softly on the table, I open the door and walk out onto the deck. Hondo's fur shines in the sunlight. He feels the vibrations of my steps and his tail begins to move slowly, back and forth.

Page Lambert

1,716 Letters

On November 15, 1942, I eagerly said "I do" to my dashing groom, who was proudly wearing his crisp, formal
United States Army uniform. Only a short eight months
later, he was called to serve in World War II, bound for an
unknown destination in the Pacific for an unknown
period of time.

When my young husband left, we made a promise to
write each other every day we were apart. We decided
we'd number each of the letters we sent so we would
know if any went astray. Writing to each other daily, we
found there were many times that there was little to say
other than "I love you." But in every single letter those
words were included.

The war found my husband, an Army dentist, right on
the front lines. Still, whether he was in the heat of battle
in the Aleutians, Okinawa, or the Philippines, he always
found some time to write every day. On occasion, he even
found time for more than just writing. When he had spare
moments, he would make me gifts of jewelry out of any
indigenous materials he could find.

During one of the lulls in battle in the Philippines, he

found time to carve a beautiful mahogany letter opener with my name, *Louise,* carefully engraved on one side of the handle, and *Philippines 1944* engraved on the other side. He told me the letter opener was to help me open my daily letters from him. More than 50 years later, that letter opener still sits on my desk and is used daily to open the mail, although none of the letters I receive today are as important as the ones I received from him during the war.

There were days and weeks when I would get no mail. Of course, that would leave me fearful about my husband's well-being—many of the men in his troop had already been killed. Inevitably though, the mail service would catch up and a slew of letters would arrive at one time. I would busy myself sorting them by number so I could read them in chronological order and savor each one. Unfortunately, every letter was screened by Army censors, and I would have to try to imagine what was written under the blacked-out lines.

In one of the letters, when my husband was in Hawaii, he asked me to send my measurements so he could have some lounging pajamas made for me by the famous Chinese tailors living on the island. So I responded by sending him my 35-24-36 measurements. (Oh, those were the good old days.) My husband received the letter but the measurements had been blacked out by the Army censors, who had thought I was trying to communicate to him by secret code. Somehow, the pajamas fit anyway.

By November 1945, the war was over and my husband was finally sent home. We had not seen each other since he had left more than two years and four months earlier. We had spoken to each other by phone only once during that entire time. But since we had faithfully kept our promise to write daily, we each had written 858 letters to each other—a total of 1,716 letters that had carried us both through the war.

When my husband returned from the war, we were fortunate to obtain a minuscule apartment in a tremendously
tight real estate market in San Francisco. In these box-like
quarters there was barely room for the two of us, so to our
regret, we had to dispose of all our letters. In the years since
the war ended, we've been fortunate to have never been
apart for more than one or two days at a time, so we've had
little opportunity to write each other letters again.

But through all the years, my husband has continued to
show me and our children and grandchildren the devotion and love he showed me in those early days. We've
just celebrated 53 years of being happily married, and
while the letters from those first few years of our marriage
no longer remain, the love within them will be forever
engraved in our hearts.

Louise Shimoff

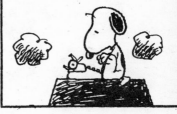

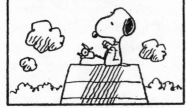

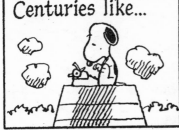

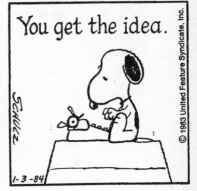

PEANUTS. *Reprinted by permission of United Feature Syndicate, Inc.*

Martha's Secret Ingredient

It bothered Ben every time he went through the kitchen. It was that little metal container on the shelf above Martha's cookstove. He probably would not have noticed it so much or been bothered by it if Martha had not repeatedly told him never to touch it. The reason, she said, was that it contained a "secret herb" from her mother, and since she had no way of ever refilling the container, she was concerned that if Ben or anyone else ever picked it up and looked inside, they might accidentally drop it and spill its valuable contents.

The container wasn't really much to look at. It was so old that much of its original red and gold floral colors had faded. You could tell right where it had been gripped again and again as the container was lifted and its tight lid pulled off.

Not only Martha's fingers had gripped it there, but her mother's and her grandmother's had, too. Martha didn't know for sure, but she felt that perhaps even her great-grandmother had used this same container and its "secret herb."

All Ben knew for sure was that shortly after he'd married

Martha, her mother had brought the container to Martha and told her to make the same loving use of its contents as she had.

And she did, faithfully. Ben never saw Martha cook a dish without taking the container off the shelf and sprinkling just a little of the "secret herb" over the ingredients. Even when she baked cakes, pies and cookies, he saw her add a light sprinkling just before she put the pans in the oven.

Whatever was in that container, it sure worked, for Ben felt Martha was the best cook in the world. He wasn't alone in that opinion—anyone who ever ate at their house grandly praised Martha's cooking.

But why wouldn't she let Ben touch that little container? Was she really afraid he'd spill its contents? And what did that "secret herb" look like? It was so fine that whenever Martha sprinkled it over the food she was preparing, Ben couldn't quite make out its texture. She obviously had to use very little of it because there was no way of refilling the container.

Somehow Martha had stretched those contents over 30 years of marriage to date. It never failed to effect mouth-watering results.

Ben became increasingly tempted to look into that container just once, but never brought himself to do so.

Then one day Martha became ill. Ben took her to the hospital, where they kept her overnight. When he returned home, he found it extremely lonely in the house. Martha had never been gone overnight before. And when it neared supper time, he wondered what to do—Martha had so loved to cook, he'd never bothered to learn much about preparing food.

As he wandered into the kitchen to see what might be in the refrigerator, the container on the shelf immediately came into view. His eyes were drawn to it like a magnet—

he quickly looked away, but his curiosity drew him back.

Curiosity nagged.

What was in that container? Why wasn't he to touch it? What did that "secret herb" look like? How much of it was left?

Ben looked away again and lifted the cover of a large cake pan on the kitchen counter. Ahh . . . there was more than half of one of Martha's great cakes left over. He cut off a large piece, sat down at the kitchen table, and hadn't taken more than one bite when his eyes went back to that container again. What would it hurt if he looked inside? Why was Martha so secretive about that container, anyway?

Ben took another bite and debated with himself—should he or shouldn't he? For five more big bites he thought about it, staring at the container. Finally he could no longer resist.

He walked slowly across the room and ever so carefully took the container off the shelf—fearing that, horror of horrors, he'd spill the contents while sneaking a peek.

He set the container on the counter and carefully pried off the lid. He was almost scared to look inside! When the inside of the container came into full view, Ben's eyes opened wide—why, the container was empty . . . except for a little folded slip of paper at the bottom.

Ben reached down for the paper, his big rugged hand struggling to get inside. He carefully picked it up by a corner, removed it and slowly unfolded it under the kitchen light.

A brief note was scrawled inside, and Ben immediately recognized the handwriting as that of Martha's mother. Very simply it said: "Martha—To everything you make, add a dash of love."

Ben swallowed hard, replaced the note and the container,

and quietly went back to finishing his cake. Now he completely understood why it tasted so good.

Submitted by Dot Abraham
Reminisce *magazine*

2

ON ATTITUDE AND SELF-ESTEEM

You don't get to choose how you're going to die or when. You can only decide how you're going to live.

Joan Baez

Be a Queen

EDITORS' NOTE: Over the years, we have been inspired by messages about love and the power of choice that great women of the world have given us. One of the most inspiring messages has come through the words, actions, and examples of one of the world's most loved and respected women, Oprah Winfrey. Continually she reminds us that within every woman lies a queen, waiting to claim her glory. Referring to a theme used by Marianne Williamson in her book *A Woman's Worth*, Oprah said the following in a commencement address to the graduates of all-female Spelman College in 1993:

> Be a queen. Dare to be different. Be a pioneer. Be a leader. Be the kind of woman who in the face of adversity will continue to embrace life and walk fearlessly toward the challenge. Take it on! Be a truth seeker and rule your domain, whatever it is—your home, your office, your family—with a loving heart.
>
> Be a queen. Be tender. Continue to give birth to new ideas and rejoice in your womanhood . . . My prayer is that we will stop wasting time being mundane and

mediocre . . . We are daughters of God—here to teach the world how to love . . .

It doesn't matter what you've been through, where you come from, who your parents are—nor your social or economic status. None of that matters. What matters is how you choose to love, how you choose to express that love through your work, through your family, through what you have to give to the world . . .

Be a queen. Own your power and your glory!

Oprah Winfrey

Home Is Where The Heart Is

Nothing had ever hit me quite so hard as driving behind the ambulance that was taking my dear friend, Alice, away to live in a nursing home. As lightening snagged the dark, rainy April morning sky, I caught a glimpse of the note Alice had scribbled back in her hospital room: *"Don't let them put me in that place!"*

But Alice had exceeded her allotted hospital stay and there was nothing I could do to stop her being moved. She was unable to breathe on her own and was connected to a ventilator, requiring complex care twenty-four hours a day. My hands were as tied as the restraints that kept Alice from pulling out her tubes when she got confused at night.

Alice had been my neighbor when I was growing up. She'd lived alone, and how she'd welcomed me into her generous heart and wonderful big red brick home. Gracious hospitality was practically a reflex for Alice. She was an art teacher and always had a jumble of creative projects going at any given moment. I loved her old-timey furnishings and the cozy clutter of her "stuff"—her "make something out of nothing" works in progress: trinkets, stacks of books, and little gifts she kept on hand for friends who happened by.

The nursing home buzzed with activity and the latest technology and even had a homey parlor, kitchen, and dining room. But it wasn't home. It was Alice's worst fear come to life. The morning she was admitted, she shook her head in despair at residents lined up in the halls in wheelchairs, like cars stopped at a red light that never turned green. Overnight, her life was reduced to a bed and a body with vacant eyes that announced, "Nobody's home anymore."

The nursing home staff, however, orchestrated an amazingly successful respiratory rehabilitation program for Alice. As the months passed, we clung to a snippet of resurrected hope that someday she might return to the home she loved so. But Alice experienced several setbacks and ran out of money for medical expenses before that could happen. Everything she'd worked so hard for had to be liquidated to pay for her care. One devastating day, the Realtor's "SOLD" sign appeared in Alice's yard. In no time, an endless parade of estate sale shoppers were sorting through her "stuff" and carrying her dearly familiar treasures away.

It was like watching a funeral procession. This is supposed to happen after you're dead, I agonized, not to someone you love who is still alive and dreaming of going home. I mourned not only for Alice's loss but for mine as well. Never again would I feel the warmth of being a guest in her home.

For weeks I couldn't bring myself to visit Alice. Grief stalked me at the oddest moments and was my constant companion in my job of styling homes for magazine photography. Then late one evening after a photo shoot at a charming Victorian cottage hear the nursing home, I dropped by to visit her. She was napping, and in the gathering blackness, her raised side rails resembled a prison cell. All of her worldly possessions were piled in bed with her—her purse, a box of tissues, partially completed sketches, stationery and pens. My eyes fell upon a big roll of address labels. They featured the address of the nursing home—not Alice's home we both loved so. I choked back tears at the finality of the situation. Plain and simple, this was to be Alice's permanent address until heaven. "Dear Lord," I prayed. "Help us both . . . somehow."

I tapped Alice's shoulder to rouse her and switched on the lamp above her tiny bed. Her tightly permed gray curls framed gentle wrinkles. "It's me—Roberta," I whispered, trying to sound cheerful.

A smile flashed across Alice's face, lighting up the darkness. It was strangely full of promise. "Let my siderail down, honey," she asked. She drew her legs in closer to make room for me, then patted the nubby pink bedspread, smoothing a spot for me to sit on the edge of the bed. I squeezed in next to her open Bible and devotional book. They were stretched out at the foot of her bed like a welcome mat. "Saved you something from my dinner tray," she said as she retrieved two vanilla wafers, tucked inside a brown paper towel, from her nightstand drawer.

"Alice, these are my favorite," I gasped. "You remembered."

"Well, look behind the curtain. I won you a little something at our party." Nestled inside a gaily wrapped box that once held medical examination gloves was a pretty pot of potpourri. Alice stirred it with her finger to release its spicy scent. "Cinnamon," she explained. "It will make your kitchen smell real good."

That afternoon, I'd sipped gourmet coffee and nibbled fancy cookies at a table dressed in antique linens and lace, finely etched crystal, and delicate china. It was picture-perfect, and in a few months it would grace the pages of a glossy decorating magazine. But it didn't come close to Alice's loving gestures, her simple sharing of everything she had. All at once, the longing in my spirit was filled with a peaceful, new understanding that when your home is in your heart, it travels with you wherever you go.

Alice and I enjoyed one of our best visits ever, reminiscing about the old neighborhood and thanking the Lord for Alice's new one. She was excited about leading a little crafts group, and I welcomed her advice about wallpapering my bedroom. When it was time for me to leave her snug room, Alice hobbled beside me down the long hallway to the front door. "They take such good care of me here," she reassured me. "Why I don't even have to find someone to mow the grass." As I headed to my car, Alice paused in the doorway, wearing the new housecoat I'd brought her. She waved and blew me a kiss. Out of the corner of my eye, I saw her chuckling with her new family.

I smiled to myself. Alice's heart was home. And thanks to answered prayer and some true hospitality, at long last, so was mine.

Roberta L. Messner

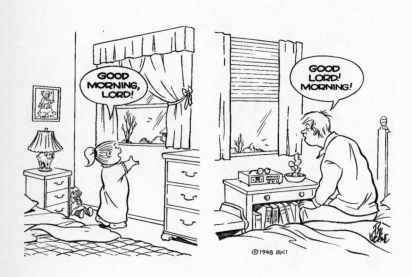

Reprinted by permission of Bil Keane.

A Tale of Two Cities

A traveler nearing a great city asked a woman seated by the wayside, "What are the people like in the city?"

"How were the people where you came from?"

"A terrible lot," the traveler responded. "Mean, untrustworthy, detestable in all respects."

"Ah," said the woman, "you will find them the same in the city ahead."

Scarcely was the first traveler gone when another one stopped and also inquired about the people in the city before him. Again the old woman asked about the people in the place the traveler had left.

"They were fine people; honest, industrious, and generous to a fault. I was sorry to leave," declared the second traveler.

Responded the wise woman: "So you will find them in the city ahead."

The Best of Bits & Pieces

Where Do the Mermaids Stand?

What is right for one soul may not be right for another. It may mean having to stand on your own and do something strange in the eyes of others.

Eileen Caddy

Giants, Wizards and Dwarfs was the game to play.

Being left in charge of about 80 children 7 to 10 years old, while their parents were off doing parenty things, I mustered my troops in the church social hall and explained the game. It's a large-scale version of Rock, Paper and Scissors, and involves some intellectual decision making. But the real purpose of the game is to make a lot of noise and run around chasing people until nobody knows which side you are on or who won.

Organizing a roomful of wired-up grade-schoolers into two teams, explaining the rudiments of the game, achieving consensus on group identity—all of this is no mean accomplishment, but we did it with a right good will and were ready to go.

The excitement of the chase had reached a critical mass. I yelled out: "You have to decide *now* which you are—a GIANT, a WIZARD or a DWARF!"

While the groups huddled in frenzied, whispered consultation, a tug came at my pant leg. A small child stands there looking up, and asks in a small concerned voice, "Where do the Mermaids stand?"

Where do the Mermaids stand?

A long pause. A *very* long pause. "Where do the Mermaids stand?" says I.

"Yes. You see, I am a Mermaid."

"There are no such things as Mermaids."

"Oh yes there is, I am one!"

She did not relate to being a Giant, a Wizard or a Dwarf. She knew her category, Mermaid, and was not about to leave the game and go over and stand against the wall where a loser would stand. She intended to participate, wherever Mermaids fit into the scheme of things, without giving up dignity or identity. She took it for granted that there was a place for Mermaids and that I would know just where.

Well, where *do* the Mermaids stand? All the Mermaids— all those who are different, who do not fit the norm, and who do not accept the available boxes and pigeonholes?

Answer that question and you can build a school, a nation or a world on it.

What was my answer at the moment? Every once in a while I say the right thing. "The Mermaid stands right here by the King of the Sea!" (Yes, right here by the King's Fool, I thought to myself.)

So we stood there hand in hand, reviewing the troops of Wizards and Giants and Dwarfs as they rolled by in wild disarray.

It is not true, by the way, that Mermaids do not exist.
I know at least one personally. I have held her hand.

Robert Fulghum
Submitted by Rashaun C. Geter

The Pirate

We don't see things as they are, we see them as we are.

Anaïs Nin

One day Mrs. Smith was sitting in her doctor's waiting room when a young boy and his mother entered the office. The young boy caught Mrs. Smith's attention because he wore a patch over one eye. She marveled at how unaffected he seemed to be by the loss of an eye and watched as he followed his mother to a chair nearby.

The doctor's office was very busy that day, so Mrs. Smith had an opportunity to chat with the boy's mother while he played with his soldiers. At first he sat quietly, playing with the soldiers on the arm of the chair. Then he silently moved to the floor, glancing up at his mother.

Eventually, Mrs. Smith had an opportunity to ask the little boy what had happened to his eye. He considered her question for a long moment, then replied, lifting the patch, "There's nothing wrong with my eye. I'm a pirate!" Then he returned to his game.

Mrs. Smith was there because she had lost her leg from the knee down in an auto accident. Her trip today was to determine whether it had healed enough to be fitted with a prosthetic. The loss had been devastating to her. Try as she would to be courageous, she felt like an invalid. Intellectually, she knew that this loss should not interfere with her life, but emotionally, she just couldn't overcome this hurdle. Her doctor had suggested visualization, and she had tried it, but had been unable to envision an emotionally acceptable, lasting image. In her mind she saw herself as an invalid.

The word "pirate" changed her life. Instantly, she was transported. She saw herself dressed as Long John Silver, standing aboard a pirate ship. She stood with her legs planted wide apart—one pegged. Her hands were clenched at her hips, her head up and her shoulders back, as she smiled into a storm. Gale force winds whipped her coat and hair behind her. Cold spray blew across the deck balustrade as great waves broke against the ship. The vessel rocked and groaned under the storm's force. Still she stood firmly—proud, undaunted.

In that moment, the invalid image was replaced and her courage returned. She regarded the young boy, busy with his soldiers.

A few minutes later, the nurse called her. As she balanced on her crutches, the young boy noticed her amputation. "Hey lady," he called, "what's wrong with your leg?" The young boy's mother was mortified.

Mrs. Smith looked down at her shortened leg for a moment. Then she replied with a smile, "Nothing. I'm a pirate, too."

Marjorie Wallé

So . . . What Do You Grow?

We are not rich by what we possess but rather by what we can do without.

Immanuel Kant

Sandy lives in an apartment so small that when she comes home from shopping at Goodwill, she has to decide what to move out to make room for her purchases. She struggles day-to-day to feed and clothe herself and her four-year-old daughter on money from freelance writing and odd jobs.

Her ex-husband has long since disappeared down some unknown highway, probably never to be heard from again. As often as not, her car decides it needs a day off and refuses to budge. That means bicycling (weather permitting), walking or bumming a ride from friends.

The things most Americans consider essential for survival—a television, microwave, boom box and high-priced sneakers—are far down Sandy's list of "maybe someday" items.

Nutritious food, warm clothing, an efficiency apartment, student loan payments, books for her daughter, absolutely necessary medical care and an occasional movie matinee eat up what little cash there is to go around.

Sandy has knocked on more doors than she can recall, trying to land a decent job, but there is always something that doesn't quite fit—too little experience or not the right kind, or hours that make child care impossible.

Sandy's story is not unusual. Many single parents and older people grapple with our economic structure, falling into the crevice between being truly self-sufficient and being sufficiently impoverished to gain government assistance.

What makes Sandy unusual is her outlook.

"I don't have much in the way of stuff or the American dream," she told me with a genuine smile.

"Does that bother you?" I asked.

"Sometimes. When I see another little girl around my daughter's age who has nice clothes and toys, or who is riding around in a fancy car or living in a fine house, then I feel bad. Everyone wants to do well by their children," she replied.

"But you're not bitter?"

"What's to be bitter about? We aren't starving or freezing to death, and I have what is really important in life," she replied.

"And what is that?" I asked.

"As I see it, no matter how much stuff you buy, no matter how much money you make, you really only get to keep three things in life," she said.

"What do you mean by 'keep'?"

"I mean that nobody can take these things away from you."

"And what are these three things?" I asked.

"One, your experiences; two, your true friends; and three, what you grow inside yourself," she told me without hesitation.

For Sandy, "experiences" don't come on a grand scale. They are so-called ordinary moments with her daughter, walks in the woods, napping under a shade tree, listening to music, taking a warm bath or baking bread.

Her definition of friends is more expansive. "True friends are the ones who never leave your heart, even if they leave your life for a while. Even after years apart, you pick up with them right where you left off, and even if they die, they're never dead in your heart," she explained.

As for what we grow inside, Sandy said, "That's up to each of us, isn't it? I don't grow bitterness or sorrow. I could if I wanted to, but I'd rather not."

"So what do you grow?" I asked.

Sandy looked warmly at her daughter and then back to me. She pointed toward her own eyes, which were aglow with tenderness, gratitude and a sparkling joy.

"I grow this."

Philip Chard
Submitted by Laurie Waldron

Grandma Ruby

Being a mother of two very active boys, ages seven and one, I am sometimes worried about their making a shambles of my carefully decorated home. In their innocence and play, they occasionally knock over my favorite lamp or upset my well-designed arrangements. In these moments when nothing feels sacred, I remember the lesson I learned from my wise mother-in-law, Ruby.

Ruby is the mother of 6 and grandmother of 13. She is the embodiment of gentleness, patience and love.

One Christmas, all the children and grandchildren were gathered as usual at Ruby's home. Just the month before, Ruby had bought beautiful new white carpeting after living with the "same old carpet" for over 25 years. She was overjoyed with the new look it gave her home.

My brother-in-law, Arnie, had just distributed his gifts for all the nieces and nephews—prized homemade honey from his beehives. They were excited. But as fate would have it, eight-year-old Sheena spilled her tub of honey on Grandma's new carpeting and trailed it throughout the entire downstairs of the house.

Crying, Sheena ran into the kitchen and into Grandma

Ruby's arms. "Grandma, I've spilled my honey all over your brand new carpet."

Grandma Ruby knelt down, looked tenderly into Sheena's tearful eyes and said, "Don't worry sweetheart, we can get you more honey."

Lynn Robertson

Problem or Solution?

It was 1933. I had been laid off my part-time job and could no longer make my contribution to the family larder. Our only income was what Mother could make by doing dressmaking for others.

Then Mother was sick for a few weeks and unable to work. The electric company came out and cut off the power when we couldn't pay the bill. Then the gas company cut off the gas. Then the water company. But the Health Department made them turn the water back on for reasons of sanitation. The cupboard got very bare. Fortunately, we had a vegetable garden and were able to cook some of its produce in a campfire in the back yard.

Then one day my younger sister came tripping home from school with, "We're supposed to bring something to school tomorrow to give to the poor."

Mother started to blurt out, "I don't know of anyone who is any poorer than we are," when her mother, who was living with us at the time, shushed her with a hand on her arm and a frown.

"Eva," she said, "if you give that child the idea that she is 'poor folks' at her age, she will be 'poor folks' for the rest of her life. There is one jar of that homemade jelly left. She can take that."

Grandmother found some tissue paper and a little bit of pink ribbon with which she wrapped our last jar of jelly, and Sis tripped off to school the next day proudly carrying her "gift to the poor."

And ever after, if there was a problem in the community, Sis just naturally assumed that she was supposed to be part of the solution.

Edgar Bledsoe

Just the Way You Are

My friend Mark Tucker produces and delivers multi-media slide presentations to audiences across the country.

One night, following one of his shows on the East Coast, a woman came up to him and said, "You know, you really should be using my son's music in your show."

So Mark started to give her the usual rap. First, her son should make a demo tape. It didn't have to be professional, he explained. In fact, her son could just go into his bedroom and play some simple chords on his guitar—just enough to give Mark an idea of the type of music he played.

After he had explained the whole process, the woman gave him a funny look and said, "Well, my son is Billy Joel."

As soon as he had recovered from the shock, Mark quickly assured her that her son would not need to send a demo tape! He then listened as this woman urged him to consider using one particular song her son had written. She felt it contained a positive message about self-worth that would fit Mark's work beautifully. And she went on to describe how the seeds of that song had been planted in early childhood.

As a young boy, she explained, Billy Joel often wanted to be someone else, someone different from who he was. It seems he was teased a lot because he was shorter than the rest of the kids. It was common for him to come home from school or play and complain that he wasn't good enough. And he truly believed that if he could be just a little taller, then he'd be okay.

His mother, of course, never believed for a minute that her son was anything less than perfect. So every time he expressed something negative about himself, she said to him, "Don't worry—it doesn't matter. You don't have to be like anyone else because you're already perfect. We're all unique, we're all different. And you, too, have something wonderful to share with the world. I love you just the way you are."

Remember that old expression about words coming back to haunt you? In this case, the words of a mother who unconditionally loved her son came back many years later in the form of a song. You see, as Billy Joel grew up, he learned who he was and he found his dream of creating music for the world. And millions of people got to hear with their hearts, as his mother did, the words of his Grammy Award-winning song:

> *Don't go changin'*
> *to try and please me . . .*
> *I love you just the way you are.*

> Jennifer Read Hawthorne

"Just the Way You Are," lyrics by Billy Joel, copyright 1977 Impulsive Music. All rights reserved. Used by permission.

True Beauty

When asked how she still appears young despite her difficult lifestyle, Mother Teresa replied, "Sometimes a good feeling from inside is worth much more than a beautician."

For Mother's Day, Jeannie had put considerable effort and planning into buying something very special for her mother, Bess. She had carefully put together the cost of an image consultation gift certificate out of her first few paychecks. On the appointed day, this young daughter brought her shy, plain mother to my studio.

During the color draping and makeover, Bess confessed that she had concentrated on her family for years and ignored herself. Consequently she had never even considered what clothes looked good on her or how to apply her makeup.

As I placed pretty colors close to her face, she began to blossom, though she didn't seem to realize it. After applying the finishing touches of blush and lipstick to enhance her coloring, I invited her to view herself in the big cheval mirror. She took a long look, as if she were surveying a stranger, then edged closer and closer to her image. Finally, staring open-mouthed, she touched the mirror lightly. "Jeannie," she motioned, "come here." Drawing her daughter beside her, she pointed toward the image. "Jeannie, look at me. I'm beautiful!"

The young woman smiled at the older woman in the mirror with tears in her eyes. "Yes, Mother, you have always been—beautiful."

Charlotte Ward

Angela's Word

When Angela was very young,
Age two or three or so,
Her mother and her father
Taught her never to say NO.
They taught her that she must agree
With everything they said,
And if she didn't, she was spanked
And sent upstairs to bed.

So Angela grew up to be
A most agreeable child;
She was never angry
And she was never wild;
She always shared, she always cared,
She never picked a fight,
And no matter what her parents said,
She thought that they were right.

Angela the Angel did very well in school
And, as you might imagine, she followed every rule;
Her teachers said she was so well-bred,
So quiet and so good,

But how Angela felt inside
They never understood.

Angela had lots of friends
Who liked her for her smile;
They knew she was the kind of gal
Who'd go the extra mile;
And even when she had a cold
And really needed rest,
When someone asked her if she'd help
She always answered Yes.

When Angela was thirty-three, she was a lawyer's wife.
She had a home and family, and a nice suburban life.
She had a little girl of four
And a little boy of nine,
And if someone asked her how she felt
She always answered, "Fine."

But one cold night near Christmastime
When her family was in bed,
She lay awake as awful thoughts went spinning through
   her head;
She didn't know why, and she didn't know how,
But she wanted her life to end;
So she begged Whoever put her here
To take her back again.

And then she heard, from deep inside,
A voice that was soft and low;
It only said a single word
And the word it said was . . . NO.

From that moment on, Angela knew
Exactly what she had to do.
Her life depended on that word,
So this is what her loved ones heard:

NO, I just don't want to;
NO, I don't agree;
NO, that's yours to handle;
NO, that's wrong for me;
NO, I wanted something else;
NO, that hurt a lot!
NO, I'm tired, and NO, I'm busy,
And NO, I'd rather not!

Well, her family found it shocking,
Her friends reacted with surprise;
But Angela was different, you could see it in her eyes;
For they've held no meek submission
Since that night three years ago
When Angela the Angel
Got permission to say NO.

Today Angela's a person first, then a mother and a wife.
She knows where she begins and ends,
She has a separate life.
She has talents and ambitions,
She has feelings, needs and goals.
She has money in the bank and
An opinion at the polls.

And to her boy and girl she says,
"It's nice when we agree;
But if you can't say NO, you'll never grow
To be all you're meant to be.
Because I know I'm sometimes wrong
And because I love you so,
You'll always be my angels
Even when you tell me NO."

Barbara K. Bassett

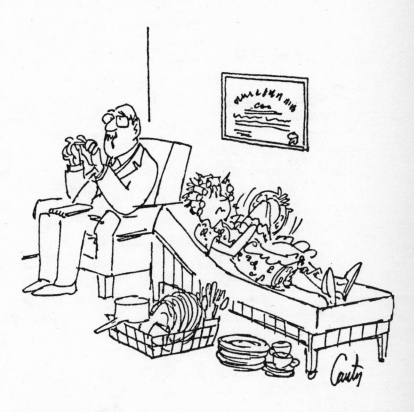

"It's imperative, Mrs. Carlson, that you put aside some time exclusively for yourself."

Reprinted with permission from William Canty.

Just Say Yes

*L*ife *is either a daring adventure or nothing at all.*

Helen Keller

I'm a standup comic. I was working at a radio station in New York, doing the weather as this character called June East (Mae West's long-lost sister). One day, a woman from *The Daily News* called and said she wanted to do an article on me. When she had finished interviewing me for the article, she asked, "What are you planning to do next?"

Well, at the time, there was absolutely nothing I was planning on doing next, so I asked her what she meant, stalling for time. She said she really wanted to follow my career. Here was a woman from *The Daily News* telling me she was interested in me! So I thought I'd better tell her something. What came out was, "I'm thinking about breaking the Guinness Book of World Records for Fastest-Talking Female."

The newspaper article came out the next day, and the writer had included my parting remarks about trying to break the world's Fastest-Talking Female record. At about

5:00 P.M. that afternoon, I got a call from *Larry King Live* asking me to go on the show. They wanted me to try to break the record, and they told me they would pick me up at 8:00—because they wanted me to do it *that night!*

Now, I had never heard of *Larry King Live,* and when I heard the woman say she was from the Manhattan Channel, I thought, *Hmmm, that's a porn channel, right?* But she patiently assured me that it was a national television show and that this was a one-time offer and opportunity—it was either that night or not at all.

I stared at the phone. I had a gig that night in New Jersey, but it wasn't hard to figure out which of the two engagements I'd prefer to do. I had to find a replacement for my 7:00 show, and I started calling every comic I knew. By the grace of God, I finally found one who would fill in for me, and five minutes before the deadline, I told *Larry King Live* I could make it.

Then I sat down to figure out what on earth I was going to do on the show. I called Guinness to find out how to break a fast-talking record. They told me I would have to recite something from either Shakespeare or the Bible.

Suddenly I started saying the ninety-first Psalm, a prayer of protection my mother had taught me. Shakespeare and I had never really gotten along, so I figured the Bible was my only hope. I began practicing and practicing, over and over again. I was both nervous and excited at the same time.

At 8:00, the limousine picked me up. I practiced the whole way there, and by the time I reached the New York studio, I was tongue-tied. I asked the woman in charge, "What if I don't break the record?"

"Larry doesn't care if you break it or not," she said. "He just cares that you try it on his show first." So I asked myself, *What's the worst that can happen? I'll look like a fool on national television! A minor thing,* I told myself, thinking

I could live through that. And what if I broke the record?

So I decided just to give it my best shot, and I did. I broke the record, becoming the World's Fastest-Talking Female by speaking 585 words in one minute in front of a national television audience. (I broke it again two years later, with 603 words in a minute.) My career took off.

People often ask me how I did that. Or how I've managed to do many of the things I've done, like lecturing for the first time, or going on stage for the first time, or bungee jumping for the first time. I tell them I live my life by this simple philosophy: I always say yes first; then I ask, *Now, what do I have to do to accomplish that?*

Then I ask myself, *What is the worst thing that can happen if I don't succeed?* The answer is, I simply don't succeed! And what's the best thing that can happen? I succeed!

What more can life ask of you? Be yourself, and have a good time!

Fran Capo

The Gift of Gab

Although she told me not to talk to strangers, my mother always did. At the checkout line. Browsing through handbags at Marshall Field. During a slow elevator ride, when everyone else was seriously squinting at the buttons. At airports, football games and the beach.

Thankfully, I only took her advice when it came to menacing strangers. I believe I'm better for it.

My mother's habit of striking up conversations with people next to her may bring a smile to my eyes now, but it proved rather embarrassing during my tender teenage years. "Lynn's getting her first one, too," she confided to a woman also shopping with her adolescent daughter in the bra section of our hometown department store. I contemplated running and hiding under a nearby terry cloth bathrobe, but instead I turned crimson and hissed "Mothhhhhherrrrr" between gritted teeth. I felt only slightly better when the girl's mother said, "We're trying to find one for Sarah, but they're all too big."

Not everyone responded when Mom made an observation and tried to spark a brief discussion. Some people gave her a tight-lipped half-grin, then turned away. A few completely ignored her. Whenever I was with her during those times, I could see that she was a little hurt, but she'd shrug it off and we'd continue on our way.

More often than not, however, I would wander off somewhere and come back to find her gabbing away. There were occasions when I was concerned that I'd lost her in the crowd, but then I'd hear her singsong laugh and a comment like, "Yes, yes, me too."

Through these spontaneous chats, my mother taught me that our world is much too large—or too small, take your pick—not to have time to reach out to one another. She reminded me that as women, we enjoy a special kind of kinship, even if we're really not all that alike. In the most mundane things, there are common threads that bind us. It may be the reason we like paper versus plastic, or why a navy sweater is never a bad buy, or why the national anthem still gives us goose bumps.

One of the last memories of my mother, when she was in the hospital and a few hours from dying from the breast cancer that had ravaged her down to 85 pounds, is of her smiling weakly and talking to her nurse about how to best plant tulip bulbs. I stood silently in the doorway, wanting to cry but feeling such a surge of love and warmth. She taught me to see spring in others. I'll never forget it, especially now when I turn to someone and say, "Don't you just love it when . . ."

Lynn Rogers Petrak

I Was a Sixth-Grade Scarecrow

*K*ind *words can be short and easy to speak, but their echoes are truly endless.*

Mother Teresa

"*Shame* on you! A *sixth-grader* and *still* acting like a god-less *heathen!*" Mrs. Brimm snarled, shoving me onto the slippery wooden bench of the principal's office. (Privately, we kids had renamed her "Mrs. Grimm." Just *my* luck she'd been on playground duty when I decided to teach my worst tormentor, Johnny Welson, a well-deserved les-son.) The fearsome third-grade teacher, her perfect, black Dutch bob swaying against geisha-white cheeks, arched penciled peaks of disapproval over flinty eyes.

How different she was from Mrs. Peterson, my stately sixth-grade teacher, who even when she was serious seemed to be on the verge of a smile. However, Mrs. Peterson was nowhere in sight. *Nobody even cares about my side!* I thought, pushing back my fear with a burst of hurt and anger. *John and those guys can give me noogies, trip me and call me names all year, and every time I start to pay someone back,* she *shows up and blames* me!

"*When* are you going to *grow up* and behave like a *young lady* . . .?" Mrs. Brimm hissed, releasing my arm at last with disgust. "You stay *here!* Miss Moss," Mrs. Brimm commanded, as the startled face of the receptionist popped timidly around a tall filing cabinet, "don't you let this juvenile delinquent out of your *sight!*" Retracting her wrinkled neck like a flustered hen, Miss Moss took one look at my mud-smeared face and Mrs. Brimm's murderous look, flapped her hands wordlessly toward the open door of the inner office, and scuttled to her desk. Striding into Mr. Swensen's room, Mrs. Brimm slammed the heavy door closed behind her, although verbal explosions like "*Absolutely* impossible!" and "*Disgraceful!*" shot through from time to time.

Miss Moss settled low behind her desk, scratching among her papers and opening and closing her drawers for no apparent reason, while I tried covertly to inspect what was left of my right upper arm. It was the same arm that John Rosse, the most popular boy in the class, and his best friend, John Welson, chose to punch when they called me "Beanpole," "Scarecrow," "Tin Mouth," "Retard," or, pointing to my heavy shoes, "The seven-league boots of Linda Legree" (a reference I actually found flattering, given Simon Legree's fearsome reputation).

I was the first to admit that I was no beauty. I had sprouted to my present unenviable height of five-foot-eight, in spite of having had polio the year before, leaving me "as scrawny as a plucked crow," as my grandma was fond of saying. Braces on both upper and lower teeth, corrective shoes and the hated glasses did nothing to improve the picture. Although I hunched my shoulders to look smaller, I was still the tallest kid in the whole school. And to top it all off, I had been held back that year—

supposedly to catch up with the missed months of school from my illness, but actually to give me a chance to redeem my outstandingly dismal school career.

My mother had great faith in Mrs. Peterson, the tall, serene sixth-grade teacher who, Mother had confided to her College Women's Club, "can do something with Linda if anyone can." Well, it was mid-November and this was the third time since school began that I'd been sent to the principal's office for fighting. Suddenly the inner door flew open and Mrs. Brimm hurtled by, trailing a final ". . . just *disgraceful!*" Tired-faced Mr. Swensen sagged in the doorway, looking far more defeated than I felt. *If Mrs. Peterson is going to do something with me,* I thought, *she'd better hurry!*

A week later, following a five-day suspension with many extra chores at home, a major two-parent scolding and a grim trip with my parents to Johnny Welson's house, where I was made to "apologize," speaking in the most unintelligible voice I could muster, I returned to school. Now I stood outside the classroom, hearing the cheerful hubbub and feeling like throwing up at the thought of seeing all the smug faces of my classmates.

A hand touched my shoulder and Mrs. Peterson's friendly voice said, "There you are! My goodness, I've missed you, Linda." I looked up into her crinkling eyes and her whole face smiled. "I've got a favor I'd like to talk to you about today during seat work," she continued, guiding me smoothly into the room. "I've been thinking that our room needs some beautification. Perhaps a mural of one of those rearing horses you sketch so often on your work? You're tall enough to make it fill the bulletin board by the window, and you could work on it during group reading or when-ever you're finished with your tasks." I smiled back, forget-ting momentarily the ordeal ahead. "Would you come over to my desk when the class settles down and I'll explain what I have in mind in more detail?" I nodded, feeling warmed and honored as always by her attention. She gave my hand a friendly little squeeze and turned away.

Alice Lee grinned and poked me as I walked by her desk. I looked down at her round, cheery face and she said softly, "Hi." Suddenly, from behind me I heard some giggles and loud whispers. "Hey, the scarecrow's back." That was Cherri. *I'll get her after school,* I thought fiercely, while my stomach clenched tight like a fist. "Retard, retard," singsonged Wardie Masterson under his breath, and John Rosse's voice came through the snickers, "How's the weather up there, Beanpole?" The laughter boiled up, scalding my whole body.

Then came another voice, resonant and musical, dousing the whispers and laughter instantly. "Beanpole?" it asked, filled with disbelief. All of us swung to stare at the source of the voice, as Mrs. Peterson, who had been leaning over Denise's diorama, straightened to her full height and turned, eyes wide and bewildered. "Did someone call our Linda a beanpole?" she asked again, incredulously. She seemed to float there, radiating a stillness that captured us all.

Our Linda! Mrs. Peterson made the words sound important, sacred, like *Our Father.* I almost stopped breathing with amazement. "Why, *I* always think of our Linda as our Powers model." Twenty-nine uncomprehending faces looked at her blankly. "Do you know about the Powers Modeling Agency in New York?" Mrs. Peterson asked, sweeping us all with her hazel gaze. As if our heads were all connected to the same string, we shook "no" in unison. New York! The other end of the universe from Ogden, Utah.

"Why, the Powers Modeling Agency has the most famous models in the world," she continued dramatically to her rapt audience. "All of their models are required to be at least six feet tall." A little gasp from the class, including me. A few pairs of eyes glanced at me appraisingly, but this time, instead of slouching at their gaze, I stood straighter, wishing for the first time in my life that I was even taller.

Mrs. Peterson's voice went on. "Do you know why these models have to be so tall?" she asked. Another slow shake of the corporate head. "Why, it's because tall women are statuesque, which makes clothing hang more beautifully." *Statuesque!* What a word. Mrs. Peterson smiled fondly around the group, melting the spell that had held us. She touched popular (but pitifully undersized) Annelle Crabtree's arm and said, "Are you ready to show me your outline now, Annelle?" and turned away.

I walked regally to my desk. The kids in the aisle, even John Rosse, hastily squeezed aside to clear a path. I had a lot of thinking to do, sketches to compile and decisions to make. Should I be a Powers Model *before* becoming a forest ranger and a veterinarian, or after? Would being world famous interfere with my living high atop a fire tower on some great mountain? I sat down in the scarred wood seat, savoring new hope for myself—statuesque! Fiery horses rared and cavorted in my mind's eye. Statuesque horses! What a magnificent mural it would be!

Linda Jessup

3

OVERCOMING OBSTACLES

The richness of the human experience would lose something of rewarding joy if there were no limitations to overcome.

Helen Keller

If There's a Will

Regis Philbin and I celebrate Mother's Day on our television program, LIVE with Regis & Kathie Lee, *by asking our viewers to write and tell us about a special mom. Each year we receive thousands of letters.*

People who would never write about themselves open their hearts about the mother they love. Here is one of those extraordinary and inspiring stories. This story is by Stacey Nasalroad.

I am my mother's third child, born when she was 20. When I was delivered, nurses took me from the room before she could see me. Her doctor gently explained that my left arm was missing, below the elbow. Then he gave her some advice: "Don't treat her any differently than the other girls. Demand more." And she did!

Even before my father left us, my mother had to go back to work to support our family. There were five of us girls in our Modesto, California, home, and we all had to help out. Once when I was about seven, I came out of the kitchen, whining, "Mom, I can't peel potatoes. I only have one hand."

Mom never looked up from sewing. "You get yourself into that kitchen and peel those potatoes," she told me.

"And don't ever use that as an excuse for anything again!"

Of course I could peel potatoes—with my good hand, while holding them down with my other arm. There was always a way, and Mom knew it. "If you try hard enough," she'd say, "you can do anything."

In second grade, our teacher lined up my class on the playground and had each of us race across the monkey bars, swinging from one high steel rod to the next. When it was my turn, I shook my head. Some kids behind me laughed. I went home crying.

That night I told Mom about it. She hugged me, and I saw her "we'll see about that" look. When she got off work the next afternoon, she took me back to school. At the deserted playground, Mom looked carefully at the bars.

"Now, pull up with your right arm," she advised. She stood by as I struggled to lift myself with my right hand until I could hook the bar with my other elbow. Day after day we practiced, and she praised me for every rung I reached.

I'll never forget the next time my class lined up at the monkey bars. Crossing the rungs, I looked down at the kids who'd made fun of me. Now they were standing with their mouths open.

It was that way with everything: instead of doing things for me, or excusing me, my mother insisted I find a way to do them myself. At times I resented her. *She doesn't know what it's like,* I thought. *She doesn't care how hard it is.* But one night, after a dance at my new junior high, I lay in bed sobbing. I could hear Mom come into my room.

"What's the matter?" she asked gently.

"Mom," I answered, weeping, "none of the boys would dance with me because of my arm."

For a long time I didn't hear anything. Then she said, "Oh, honey, someday you'll be beating those boys off with a bat. You'll see." Her voice was faint and cracking. I peeked out from my covers to see tears running down her cheeks. Then I knew how much she suffered on my behalf. She had never let me see her tears, though, because she didn't want me to feel sorry for myself.

Later, I married the first guy I thought accepted me. But he turned out to be immature and irresponsible. When my daughter Jessica was born, I wanted to protect her from my unhappy marriage, and I broke free.

During the five years I was a single mother, Mom was my rock. If I needed to cry, she'd hold me. If I complained about chasing a toddler around after working and going to school, she'd laugh. But if I ever started feeling sorry for myself, I'd look at her and then remember, *She did it with five!*

I remarried, and my husband Tim and I have a loving family that includes four children. Perhaps because Mom missed so much time with her own kids, she made it up with her grandchildren. Many times I watched her rock Jessica, stroking her hair. "I'm going to spoil her rotten and then give her back to her mama for some discipline," she'd tell me. "That's my privilege now." She didn't, though. She just gave the children infinite patience and love.

In 1991, Mom was found to have lung cancer and given six months to a year to live. She was still with us more than three years later. Doctors said it was a miracle; I think it was her love for her grandchildren that kept her fighting right up to the last. Mom died five days after her 53rd birthday. Even now, it hurts me to think that someone who had so much hardship in life should have suffered so at the end.

But she taught me the answer to that, too. As a child, I wondered why I had to struggle so. Now I know—it's hardship that makes us the people we become. I feel Mom with me always. Sometimes, when I fear I can't handle things, I see her radiant smile again. She had the heart to face anything. And she taught me I could, too.

Kathie Lee Gifford and Stacey Nasalroad

We've Come a Long Way

A woman is like a tea bag: You never know her strength until you drop her in hot water.
Eleanor Roosevelt

In 1996, we women are generally as solidly into networking and supporting each other as our male counterparts have been for decades. It is a much friendlier place for women than it was 40 or 50 years ago. Whenever I get complacent about that, I think about my mother—and I wonder if I could have survived what she went through back then.

By 1946, when my mother, Mary Silver, had been married to Walter Johnson for nearly seven years, she was the mother of four active, noisy children. I was the oldest, at nearly six; the others followed close behind: two boys, ages four and two, and then a girl, still just an infant. We lived in a very old house with no close neighbors.

I know little of my parents' lives at this time, but having raised two children myself in some remote corners of the country, I can imagine what it must have been like, especially for my mother. With four small children, a husband whose sense of obligation extended to bringing home the bacon and mowing the yard, no neighbors and almost no opportunities to develop any friends of her own, she had virtually no place to vent the intense pressures that must have built up in her. For some reason, my father decided that she was "straying." When she could possibly have found the time and whom she'd have been able to meet, let alone "stray" with, since the four of us were constantly underfoot, is a mystery to me. But my father made up his mind, and that was that.

One early spring day in 1946, my mother left the house to get milk for the baby. When she came back, my father was standing at an upstairs window with a gun. He said, "Mary, if you try to come into this house, I'll shoot your children." That was how he let her know that he was suing her for divorce.

That was the last time my mother ever saw that house. She was forced to walk away with only the clothes she was wearing and the money in her purse—and a quart of milk. Today, she would probably have options: a local shelter, an 800 number to call, a network of friends she had developed through a full- or part-time job. She'd have a checkbook and credit cards in her pocket. And she could turn without shame to her family for support. But in 1946, she had none of that. Married people just didn't get divorced.

So there she was—completely alone. My father had actually managed to turn her own father against her. Now my grandfather forbade my grandmother to speak to her daughter when her daughter needed her most.

At some point before they went to court, my father contacted her and said: "Look, Mary, I don't really want a divorce. I only did all this to teach you a lesson." But my mother could see that bad though her situation was, it was preferable to going back to my father and letting him raise us kids. So she said in effect, "No way. I've come this far, there's no going back."

Where could she go? There was no going home. She couldn't stay there in Amherst, first because she knew no one would take her in; second, because with the returning GIs there would be no hope of work for her; and finally, and most important, because my father was there. So she got on a bus to the only place that held any hope for her— New York City.

My mother had one thing going for her: She was well-educated, with a degree in mathematics from Mt. Holyoke College. But she had taken the usual route of women in the 1930s and '40s: She had gone directly from high school to college to marriage. She had no idea how to find work and support herself.

New York City had several things in its favor: It was only 200 miles away, so she could afford a bus ticket, and it was a big city, so there had to be a job hiding there somewhere. She absolutely had to find a way to support all four of us kids. Upon arriving in New York she located a YWCA where she could stay for $1.50 a night. There was a Horn & Hardart Automat nearby where she could put nickels into slots next to windows with food behind them, and for about $1 a day, feed herself egg salad sandwiches and coffee. Next she started pounding the streets.

For several days, which became several weeks, she found nothing: no jobs for math majors, male *or* female, no jobs for women at all. Each night she went back to the Y, washed out her underwear and her white blouse, hung them to dry, and in the morning used the Y's iron and ironing board to press the wrinkles out of the blouse. These items, along with a gray flannel skirt, constituted her entire wardrobe. Caring for them took up a portion of the long evenings she faced alone at the Y. With no books, no extra nickels or dimes for a newspaper, no telephone (and no one to call if she'd had one), and no radio except downstairs (where the Y guest list was somewhat frightening), the nights must have been truly awful.

Predictably, her money dwindled, as did the list of employment agencies. It came down finally to a particular Thursday, the last employment agency in the city, and less in her pocket than the $1.50 she needed for that night's lodging. She was trying very hard not to think about spending the night in the street.

She trudged up several flights of stairs to reach the agency, filled out the obligatory forms, and when it was her turn to be interviewed, steeled herself for the bad news. "We're really sorry, but we don't have anything for you. We hardly have jobs enough for the men we have to place." For, of course, the men came first for any available jobs.

My mother felt nothing as she rose from her chair and turned to the door. Numb as she was, she was almost out the door before she realized the woman had mumbled something else.

"I'm sorry, I missed that. What did you say?" she asked.

"Well, I said there's always George B. Buck, but nobody ever wants that job. Nobody ever stays there," the woman repeated, nodding her head toward a box of file cards on top of a nearby cabinet.

"What is it? Tell me about it," my mother said anxiously, sitting back down in the wooden chair. "I'll take anything. When does it start?"

"Well, it's a job as an actuarial clerk, which you're qualified for, but the pay's not good and I'm sure you wouldn't like it," said the agent, pulling the relevant card out of the file box. "Let's see, it says here that you can start anytime. I suppose that means you could go down there now. The morning's not too far gone."

My mother says she literally snatched the card from the agent's hand and ran down the stairs. She didn't even

stop to catch her breath as she ran the several blocks to
the address listed on the card. When she presented herself to the surprised personnel manager, he decided that
she could indeed start work that very morning if she
wanted to—there was plenty to do. And it turned out
that Thursday was payday. Back in those days most companies paid their employees out of the till for time
worked up to and including payday itself—so, miracu-
lously, when five o'clock came, she was handed cash for
the five hours she had worked that very day. It wasn't
much, but it got her through to the next Thursday, and
then the next, and so on.

Mary Silver Johnson remained with George B. Buck &
Company for 38 years, rising to a position of great respect
in the company. I remember she had a corner office—no
mean feat in downtown Manhattan. After she'd been
there 10 years, she was able to buy us a house in suburban New Jersey, half a block from a bus to the city.

These days, every second household seems to be
headed by a working single mother, and it is easy to forget that there was once a time that such a life was almost
unthinkable. I am both humbled to reflect on my mother's
accomplishments and proud enough to bust my buttons!
If I've come a long way, baby, it's because I was carried a
large part of that way by the efforts of many, many other
women before me—with this remarkable woman, my
mother, leading the way.

Pat Bonney Shepherd

And Justice Has Been Served

Life was not easy when little Sandra was a child on the lazy B Ranch. She grew up in the 1930s in a little adobe house on the Texas New Mexico border, with no electricity and no running water. With such limited resources, anyone would have thought that Sandra's future was not bright. But her parents had a dream for her—a dream that she would one day go to college, something neither of them had gotten the opportunity to do.

This would not be an easy dream for her parents to realize. First, there wasn't even a school within driving distance. So Sandra's mom, Ada Mae, began home schooling her at age four. They would read together hour after hour, day after day. And then there was the question of money. Sandra's father, Harry, had to work very hard on the family ranch to make the money they needed to be able to send her to college.

Eventually, Sandra not only went to college, but then on to law school. And in 1952 she graduated near the top of her class from Stanford University Law School. Her parents' dream had come true.

The world was now her oyster, and Sandra set out

confidently to get her first job as a lawyer. But this was 1952, and Sandra was a woman. The only offers that came her way were for jobs as a legal secretary. Though she was disappointed, she persisted and finally got her first job as a lawyer—as the assistant county attorney for San Mateo, California. Over the years, she continued to work hard, and ultimately she built a prominent law practice in Arizona.

It was 29 years after her graduation from Stanford Law School that she got the call from Attorney General William French Smith. Many years earlier, Mr. Smith had been one of the partners at a big Los Angeles law firm that had turned her down for a job as an attorney. But on that day, he was not calling to offer her a job as a legal secretary. Instead, he was calling to tell her that President Reagan had just nominated her—Sandra Day O'Connor—to be the first female justice of the U.S. Supreme Court.

Adapted from Bits & Pieces

No Hair Day

If you are turning 16, you stand in front of the mirror scrutinizing every inch of your face. You agonize that your nose is too big and you're getting another pimple— on top of which you are feeling dumb, your hair isn't blonde and that boy in your English class has not noticed you yet.

Alison never had those problems. Two years ago, she was a beautiful, popular and smart eleventh-grader, not to mention a varsity lacrosse goalie and an ocean life-guard. With her tall slender body, pool-blue eyes and thick blonde hair, she looked more like a swimsuit model than a high school student. But during that summer, something changed.

After a day of lifeguarding, Alison couldn't wait to get home, rinse the saltwater out of her hair and comb through the tangles. She flipped her sun-bleached mane forward. "Ali!" her mother cried. "What did you do?" She had discovered a bare patch of skin on the top of her daughter's scalp. "Did you shave it? Could someone else have done it when you were sleeping?" Quickly, they solved the mystery—Alison must have wrapped the elastic band too tightly around her pony tail. The incident was soon forgotten.

Three months later, another bald spot was found, then another. Soon, Alison's scalp was dotted with peculiar quarter-sized bare patches. After diagnoses of "It's just stress" to remedies of topical ointments, a specialist began to administer injections of cortisone, 50 in each spot to be exact, every two weeks. To mask her scalp, bloody from the shots, Alison was granted permission to wear a baseball hat to school, normally a violation of the strict uniform code. Little strands of hair would push through the scabs, only to fall out two weeks later. She was suffering from a condition of hair loss known as alopecia, and nothing would stop it.

Alison's sunny spirit and supportive friends kept her going, but there were some low points. Like the time when her little sister came into her bedroom with a towel wrapped around her head to have her hair combed. When her mother untwisted the towel, Alison watched the tousled thick hair bounce around her sister's shoulders. Gripping all of her limp hair between two fingers, she burst into tears. It was the first time she had cried since the whole experience began.

As time went on, a bandanna replaced the hat, which could no longer conceal her balding scalp. With only a handful of wispy strands left, the time had come to buy a wig. Instead of trying to resurrect her once long blonde hair, pretending like nothing was ever lost, she opted for an auburn shoulder-length one. Why not? People cut and dye their hair all the time. With her new look, Alison's confidence strengthened. Even when the wig blew off from an open window of her friend's car, they could all share in the humor.

As summer approached, Alison began to worry. If she couldn't wear a wig in the water, how could she lifeguard again? "Why, did you forget how to swim?" her father asked. She got the message.

And after wearing an uncomfortable bathing cap for only one day, she mustered up the courage to go completely bald. Despite the stares and occasional comments from less than polite beachcombers—"Why do you crazy punk kids shave your heads?"—Alison adjusted to her new look.

She arrived back at school that fall, no hair, no eyebrows, no eyelashes, with her wig tucked away somewhere at the back of her closet. As she had always planned, she would run for school president—changing her campaign speech only slightly. Presenting a slide show on famous bald leaders from Gandhi to Mr. Clean, Alison had the students and faculty rolling in the aisles.

In her first speech as the elected president, Alison addressed her condition, quite comfortable answering questions. Dressed in a tee shirt with the words "Bad Hair Day" printed across the front, she pointed to her shirt and said, "When most of you wake up in the morning and don't like how you look, you may put on this tee shirt." Putting on another tee shirt over the other, she continued. "When I wake up in the morning, I put on this one." It read, "No Hair Day." Everybody cheered and applauded. And Alison, beautiful, popular and smart, not to mention varsity goalie, ocean lifeguard and now school president with the pool-blue eyes, smiled back from the podium.

Alison Lambert with Jennifer Rosenfeld

Just Like You

By the time I was a junior in high school, two very important things had happened in my life. The first was that I'd fallen in love with a young man named Charlie. He was a senior, he was a football player, he was great! I *knew* that this was the young man I wanted to marry and have children with. Unfortunately, there was a serious problem: Charlie didn't know I existed. Nor did he know that we had plans!

The second important thing was that I decided I did not want any more surgeries on my hands. I was born with six fingers on each hand and no knuckles. I had started having surgery on my hands when I was six months old, and had 27 surgeries by the time I was 16. The surgeons had taken away the extra fingers, shortened some fingers and created knuckles. I had been a young specimen paraded at times in front of up to 500 hand surgeons. While my hands were still not "normal," I was done.

At 16, I figured I had the right to say, "Leave my body alone!" My family supported my decision, telling me I could have more surgeries as an adult. But I thought,

Nope. I don't need any more. This is how my hands will be. And that was that.

Growing up, I had a friend named Don. We had gone to school together since first grade, and we were really good buddies. One afternoon, Don came over to my house and we started talking about the junior-senior prom that was coming up, and our plans to stay out all night on prom night. We had no idea what we were going to *do* all night, but we were very excited about staying out.

Out of the blue, Don looked at me and said, "You really like Charlie a lot, don't you?"

I answered, "Yeah, I really do."

"But you know, Carol, there's a problem—Charlie is never going to want you," Don continued.

"Why not?" I asked. *I know—I'll dye my hair blond,* I thought to myself. *I know how that works. No, I know—I'll become a cheerleader. Everybody wants cheerleaders.*

But Don said, "Carol, you really don't understand. Charlie is never going to want you because you are deformed."

I heard it. I believed it. I lived it.

His words struck me. I became a first-grade teacher because I thought that would be a good place for someone with a deformity.

My first year teaching, I had a little girl in my classroom named Felicia. She was the most gorgeous little girl I'd ever seen in my life. One afternoon, we were all working on learning to write our A's. To a first-grader that means a big fat red pencil, lined green paper and a concentrated effort to move the pencil "all-the-way-around-and-pull-down." The classroom was very quiet as everyone worked diligently.

I looked over at Felicia as I did so often, and I saw that she was writing with her fingers crossed. I tiptoed over to her, bent down and whispered, "Felicia, why are you writing with your fingers crossed?" This little girl looked up at me with her enormous, beautiful eyes, and she said, "Because, Mrs. Price, I want to be *just like you.*"

Felicia never saw a deformity, only a specialness she wanted for herself. Every one of us has something we consider to be *not okay*—to be a deformity. We can consider ourselves deformed or we can see ourselves as special. And that choice will determine how we live our lives.

Carol Price

Little Red Wagons

To be perfectly honest, the first month was blissful. When Jeanne, Julia, Michael—ages six, four and three—and I moved from Missouri to my hometown in northern Illinois the very day of my divorce, I was just happy to find a place where there was no fighting or abuse.

But after the first month, I started missing my old friends and neighbors. I missed our lovely, modern, ranch-style brick home in the suburbs of St. Louis, especially after we'd settled into the 98-year-old white wood-frame house we'd rented, which was all my "post-divorce" income could afford.

In St. Louis we'd had all the comforts: a washer, dryer, dishwasher, TV and car. Now we had none of these. After the first month in our new home, it seemed to me that we'd gone from middle-class comfort to poverty-level panic.

The bedrooms upstairs in our ancient house weren't even heated, but somehow the children didn't seem to notice. The linoleum floors, cold on their little feet, simply encouraged them to dress faster in the mornings and to hop into bed quicker in the evenings.

I complained about the cold as the December wind whistled under every window and door in that old frame house. But the children giggled about "the funny air places" and simply snuggled under the heavy quilts Aunt Bernadine brought over the day we moved in.

I was frantic without a TV. "What will we do in the evenings without our favorite shows?" I asked. I felt cheated that the children would miss out on all the Christmas specials. But my three little children were more optimistic and much more creative than I. They pulled out their games and begged me to play Candyland and Old Maid with them.

We cuddled together on the tattered gray sofa the landlord provided and read picture book after picture book from the public library. At their insistence we played records, sang songs, popped popcorn, created magnificent Tinkertoy towers and played hide-and-go-seek in our rambling old house. The children taught me how to have fun without a TV.

One shivering December day just a week before Christmas, after walking the two miles home from my temporary part-time job at a catalog store, I remembered that the week's laundry had to be done that evening. I was dead tired from lifting and sorting other people's Christmas presents and somewhat bitter, knowing that I could barely afford any gifts for my own children.

As soon as I picked up the children from the babysitter's, I piled four large laundry baskets full of dirty clothes into their little red wagon, and the four of us headed toward the Laundromat three blocks away.

Inside, we had to wait for washing machines and then for people to vacate the folding tables. The sorting, washing, drying and folding took longer than usual.

Jeanne asked, "Did you bring any raisins or crackers, Mommy?"

"No. We'll have supper as soon as we get home," I snapped.

Michael's nose was pressed against the steamy glass window. "Look, Mommy! It's snowing! Big flakes!"

Julia added, "The street's all wet. It's snowing in the air but not on the ground!"

Their excitement only upset me more. As if the cold wasn't bad enough, now we had snow and slush to contend with. I hadn't even unpacked the box with their boots and mittens yet.

At last the clean folded laundry was stacked into the laundry baskets and placed two baskets deep in the little red wagon. It was pitch dark outside. Six-thirty already? No wonder they were hungry! We usually ate at five.

The children and I inched our way into the cold winter evening and slipped along the slushy sidewalk. Our procession of three little people, a crabby mother and four baskets of fresh laundry in an old red wagon moved slowly as the frigid wind bit our faces.

We crossed the busy four-lane street at the crosswalk. When we reached the curb, the front wagon wheels slipped on the ice and tipped the wagon over on its side, spilling all the laundry into a slushy black puddle.

"Oh no!" I wailed. "Grab the baskets, Jeanne! Julia, hold the wagon! Get back up on the sidewalk, Michael!"

I slammed the dirty wet clothes back into the baskets.

"I hate this!" I screamed. Angry tears spilled out of my eyes. I hated being poor with no car and no washer or dryer. I hated the weather. I hated being the only parent who claimed responsibility for my three small children. And without a doubt, I really hated the whole blasted Christmas season.

When we reached our house I unlocked the door, threw my purse across the room and stomped off to my bedroom for a good cry.

I sobbed loudly enough for the children to hear. Selfishly, I wanted them to know how miserable I was. Life couldn't get any worse. The laundry was still dirty, we were all hungry and tired, there was no supper started, and no outlook for a brighter future.

When the tears finally stopped, I sat up and stared at a wooden plaque of Jesus hanging on the wall at the foot of my bed. I'd had that plaque since I was a small child and had carried it with me to every house I'd ever lived in. It showed Jesus with his arms outstretched over the earth, obviously solving the problems of the world.

I kept looking at his face, expecting a miracle. I looked and waited and finally said aloud, "God, can't you do something to make my life better?"

I desperately wanted an angel on a cloud to come down and rescue me.

But nobody came . . . except Julia, who peeked in my bedroom door and told me in her tiniest four-year-old voice that she had set the table for supper.

I could hear six-year-old Jeanne in the living room sorting the laundry into two piles, "really dirty, sorta clean, really dirty, sorta clean."

Three-year-old Michael popped into my room and gave me a picture of the first snow that he had just colored.

And you know what? At that very moment I *did* see not one, but three angels before me: three little cherubs eternally optimistic, and once again pulling me from gloom and doom into the world of "things will be better tomorrow, Mommy."

Christmas that year was magical as we surrounded ourselves with a very special kind of love, based on the joy of doing simple things together. One thing's for sure: Single parenthood was never again as frightening or as depressing as it was the night the laundry fell out of the little red wagon. Those three Christmas angels have kept my spirits buoyed; and even today, over 20 years later, they continue to fill my heart with the presence of God.

Patricia Lorenz

My Father's Lessons

My father was one of those old-fashioned country preachers who spouted verses from the pulpit of his little Baptist church and made the listeners tremble in their seats. He could recite whole chapters from John without ever glancing at the Bible clutched in his hand.

One afternoon after school, my father and I drove down an old dirt road to visit one of the elderly ladies of the congregation. I had just received my new third-grade reader. It was my first real hardcover book and I was very proud of it. I had already read one story to my father and was starting another one, when I came to a word that I did not know. I held the book up so Father could see it and asked him what the word was. He mumbled something about not being able to read and drive at the same time, so very slowly I spelled the word: "a-u-t-u-m-n." My father drove on in silence. Angry, I yelled at him, "Can't you read?"

My father pulled the car over to the side of the road and turned off the ignition. "No, Cathy, I can't read," he whispered softly. "No, I can't read." He reached over and took my new book out of my hand. "I can't read anything in this book," he said with such pain that even I, an eight-year-old child, could feel it.

Very quietly, my father began to talk of his childhood, of the big family that survived by the physical labor of its members. If it was time to harvest the crops, school and books could wait. They had to hoe cotton in the summer and pick it in the fall. In the winter, they had to slaughter and preserve animals. There were many mouths to feed, and everyone had to pull his or her load. To make life even more difficult, my father had two brothers who were handicapped, so the others had to double up and do the work they could not. As a result of his excessive absences from school, my father failed several grades. His motivation to learn evaporated, and at the age of 16, he dropped out.

I will never forget the sorrow in my father's voice as he told me this story. He seemed so ashamed and saddened to not have been able to help his five children with their lessons in school.

"But Father, how could you read whole chapters of the Bible aloud from the pulpit, without ever missing a word?" I asked. He explained that he memorized the passages that my mother read aloud to him over and over. When I heard that, I loved my father more than ever. He was a remarkable man and it was at that moment that I vowed to teach him how to read.

Whatever lessons my teacher gave me at school, I shared with my father. I taught him the sounds and patterns of language as I learned them. When I read a story at school, I came home and taught my father to read it. When I struggled with a new concept, he struggled along with me. In return, he helped me find mnemonic devices to memorize items that I needed to pass tests. Soon he learned to write simple stories and poems. Then he was able to write quotations and jot down notes that he needed for his sermons. The proudest moment of my life came when my father read the scripture—really read it—for his Sunday sermon.

In 1977 doctors diagnosed my father with terminal lung cancer, and he died nine months later. During those final months, he read the Bible from Genesis through Revelation. His proudest moment was when he closed the Bible, knowing he could read all that was written inside it.

Before my father died, he thanked me for the gift that I had given him. He didn't realize, however, the gift that he had given me: I knew that just as he was called to be a pastor, I was called to be a reading teacher. Because of my father, I believe that if I can spare one child the heartache and humiliation of illiteracy, my career as a teacher is wholly worthwhile. Thank you, Father.

Cathy Downs

Who to Believe?

My doctors told me I would never walk again.
My mother told me I would. I believed my mother.

Wilma Rudolph

Let me tell you about a little girl who was born into a very poor family in a shack in the backwoods of Tennessee. She was the 20th of 22 children, prematurely born and frail. Her survival was doubtful. When she was four years old, she had double pneumonia and scarlet fever—a deadly combination that left her with a paralyzed and useless left leg. She had to wear an iron leg brace. Yet she was fortunate in having a mother who encouraged her.

Well, this mother told her little girl, who was very bright, that despite the brace and leg, she could do whatever she wanted to do with her life. She told her that all she needed to do was to have faith, persistence, courage and an indomitable spirit.

So at nine years of age, the little girl removed the leg brace and took the step the doctors told her she would never take normally. In four years, she developed a rhythmic stride, which was a medical wonder. Then this girl got the notion, the incredible notion, that she would like to be the world's greatest woman runner. Now, what could she mean—be a runner with a leg like that?

At age 13, she entered a race. She came in last—way, way last. She entered every race in high school, and in every race she came in last. Everyone begged her to quit. However, one day, she came in next to last. And then there came a day when she won a race. From then on, Wilma Rudolph won every race that she entered.

Wilma went to Tennessee State University, where she met a coach named Ed Temple. Coach Temple saw the indomitable spirit of the girl, that she was a believer and that she had great natural talent. He trained her so well that in 1960 she went to the Olympic Games in Rome.

There she was pitted against the greatest woman runner of the day, a German girl named Jutta Heine. Nobody had ever beaten Jutta. But in the 100-meter dash, Wilma Rudolph won. She beat Jutta again in the 200 meters. Wilma had just earned two Olympic gold medals.

Finally came the 400-meter relay. It would be Wilma against Jutta once again. The first two runners on Wilma's team made perfect hand-offs with the baton. But when the third runner handed the baton to Wilma, she was so excited she dropped it, and Wilma saw Jutta taking off down the track. It was impossible that anybody could catch this fleet and nimble girl. But Wilma did just that! Wilma Rudolph had earned her third Olympic gold medal.

That day she made history as she became the first woman ever to win three gold medals in the same Olympic games. And they'd said she would never walk again . . .

More Sower's Seeds

The Marks of Life

My teammates on the United States Disabled Ski Team used to tease me about the size of my chest, joking that my greatest handicap wasn't my missing leg but my missing cleavage. Little did they know how true that would become. This past year, I found out that for the second time in my life I had cancer, this time in both breasts. I had bilateral mastectomies.

When I heard I'd need the surgery, I didn't think it would be a big deal. I even told my friends playfully, "I'll keep you abreast of the situation." After all, I had lost my leg to my first go-round with cancer at age 12, then gone on to become a world-champion ski racer. All of us on the Disabled Ski Team were missing one set of body parts or another. I saw that a man in a wheelchair can be utterly sexy. That a woman who has no hands can appear not to be missing anything. That wholeness has nothing to do with missing parts and everything to do with spirit. Yet although I knew this, I was surprised to discover how difficult it was to adjust to my new scars.

When they brought me back to consciousness after the surgery, I started to sob and hyperventilate. Suddenly I found that I didn't want to face the loss of more of my body. I didn't want chemotherapy again. I didn't want to be brave and tough and put on a perpetual smiling face. I didn't ever want to wake up again. My breathing grew so shaky that the anesthesiologist gave me oxygen and then, thankfully, put me back to sleep.

When I was doing hill sprints to prepare for my ski racing—my heart and lungs and leg muscles all on fire—I'd often be hit by the sensation that there were no resources left inside me with which to keep going. Then I'd think about the races ahead—my dream of pushing my potential as far as it could go, the satisfaction of breaking through my own barriers—and that would get me through the sprints. The same tenacity that served me so well in ski racing helped me survive my second bout with cancer.

After the mastectomies, I knew that one way to get myself going would be to start exercising again, so I headed for the local pool. In the communal shower, I found myself noticing other women's breasts for the first time in my life. Size-D breasts and size-A breasts, sagging breasts and perky breasts. Suddenly and for the first time, after all these years of missing a leg, I felt acutely self-conscious. I couldn't bring myself to undress.

I decided it was time to confront myself. That night at home, I took off all my clothes and had a long look at the woman in the mirror. She was androgynous. Take my face—without makeup, it was a cute young boy's face. My shoulder muscles, arms and hands were powerful and muscular from the crutches. I had no breasts; instead, there were two prominent scars on my chest. I had a sexy flat stomach, a bubble butt and a well-developed thigh from years of ski racing. My right leg ended in another long scar just above the knee.

I discovered that I liked my androgynous body. It fit my personality—my aggressive male side that loves getting dressed in a helmet, arm guards and shin protectors to do battle with the slalom gates, and my gentle female side that longs to have children one day and wants to dress up in a beautiful silk dress, go out to dinner with a lover and then lie back and be slowly undressed by him.

I found that the scars on my chest and my leg *were* a big deal. They were my marks of life. All of us are scarred by life; it's just that some of those scars show more clearly than others. Our scars do matter. They tell us that we have lived, that we haven't hidden from life. When we see our scars plainly, we can find in them, as I did that day, our own unique beauty.

The next time I went to the pool I showered naked.

Diana Golden

Soaring Free

It is not easy to find happiness in ourselves, and impossible to find it elsewhere.

Agnes Repplier

A new home, a swimming pool in the back yard, two nice cars in the driveway and my first child on the way. After nine years of marriage I had it all—or so I thought.

I was only days away from delivering my first child when a conversation with my husband shattered the world I lived in. "I want to be here for the baby, but I don't think I love you any more," he said. I couldn't believe what I was hearing! He had grown distant during my pregnancy, but I had related it to his fear and concern over becoming a parent.

As I probed him for explanations, he told me he'd had an affair five years earlier and hadn't felt the same about me since. Thinking only of my baby, and wanting so desperately to save my marriage, I told him I could forgive him for anything and that I wanted to work things out.

That final week before my son was born was an emotional roller-coaster ride. I was so excited about the baby, so scared that I was losing my husband, and feeling so guilty at times because I thought it was the baby's fault that all this was happening.

T. J. was born on a Friday in July. He was so beautiful and so innocent. He had no idea what was happening in his mother's world. He was four weeks old when I discovered the real reason for his father's distance. Not only had he had an affair five years earlier, but he had started another affair during my pregnancy that was continuing. So T. J. and I left the new home, the swimming pool and all of my broken dreams behind when he was five weeks old. We moved into an apartment across town.

I sank to depths of depression that I hadn't known existed. I had never before experienced anything like the loneliness of spending hour after hour alone with a newborn infant. Some days the responsibility of it all overwhelmed me and I would shake with fright. Family and friends were there to help, yet there were so many hours filled with thoughts of broken dreams and despair.

I cried often, yet I made sure that T. J. never saw me cry. I was determined this wasn't going to affect him. From somewhere inside I always found a smile for him.

The first three months of T. J.'s life passed in a blur of tears. I went back to work and tried to hide from everyone what was going on. I was ashamed, though I don't know why.

It was a Saturday morning when T. J. was four months old that I hit the bottom. I had just had yet another emotional discussion with my husband and he had stormed out of my apartment. T. J. was sleeping in his crib and I found myself sitting on the bathroom floor, curled up in a ball, rocking back and forth. I heard myself say out loud, "I don't want to live anymore." After saying it, the silence was overwhelming.

I believe God was there with me that day. After saying it, I sat there in silence for a while, letting the tears flow down my cheeks. I don't know how much time passed, but from somewhere within me arose a strength I hadn't felt before. I decided then and there to take control of my life. I was no longer going to give my husband the power to affect my life in such a negative way. I realized that by focusing so much of my attention on his weaknesses, I was allowing those weaknesses to ruin my life.

That very same day, I packed a suitcase for T. J. and myself and we went to spend the weekend at my brother's house. It was the first trip I'd taken by myself with T. J., and I felt so strong and so independent! I remember on the two-hour drive I laughed, talked and sang to T. J. all the way. It was during that trip that I realized what a savior my son had been to me during all those months. Knowing that he was there every day and that he needed me had kept me going and given me a reason for getting out of bed in the morning. What a blessing he was in my life!

From that day forward, I forced myself to focus on the confidence and strength that had brought me up from the bathroom floor. Having changed my focus to such positive thoughts, I couldn't believe the difference it made in my life. I felt like laughing again and I enjoyed being around people for the first time in months. I began the process of discovering the individual I had kept hidden inside myself for so long—a process that I am still enjoying today.

I had entered counseling shortly after T. J. and I moved out of the house, and I continued in that counseling for several months after the day I felt I had hit bottom. When I no longer felt the need for her support and guidance, I remember the last question my counselor asked me before I left her office that day. "What have you learned?" she asked. I didn't even hesitate in answering. "I've learned that my happiness has to come from within."

It is this lesson that I am reminded of every day and that I long to share with others. I had made the mistake in my life of basing my identity on my marriage and all the material things surrounding that relationship. I've learned that I am responsible for my own life and happiness. When I focus my life on another person and try to build my life and happiness around that person, I'm not truly living. To truly live I need to let the spirit within me be free and rejoice in its uniqueness. It is in this state of being that the love of another person becomes a joy and not something to be afraid of losing.

May *your* spirit be free and soar high!

Laurie Waldron

Tears of Joy

Love yourself first and everything else falls into line. You really have to love yourself to get anything done in this world.

Lucille Ball

To cry is uniquely human, to weep for joy even more so. I cry every day.

I cry for all the years I wanted and needed to cry and didn't. I cry for the loneliness and pain I've felt. I cry for the sheer delight of being alive. I cry for the pleasure that moving my body brings, and for the ability to dance and stretch and sweat. I cry in gratitude for the life I have now.

I was a cute little girl. I loved laughing and playing with my friends. Then, when I was eight years old, I experienced the devastating trauma of incest. In order to cope with that physical, mental and emotional nightmare, I made two unconscious decisions: First, I wanted to be as ugly as possible; second, I didn't want to think or feel. I knew if I let myself feel anything, it would be too much for me.

So I started eating. When the fear came, I ate; when the pain came, I ate. By the time I was 12, I weighed 200 pounds.

I spent most of my time by myself, doing things with my hands or watching TV. Even with my brothers and sisters, I felt alone. I was never asked out to a dance or to a movie or on a date. I was socially invisible.

By the time I was 25, I weighed 420 pounds. My doctor gave me six months to live. My body couldn't support the fat I was carrying. I didn't leave my house for two years. I literally couldn't move. I *had* to lose the weight if I wanted to live. And I decided I would do whatever the doctor told me to do to lose it.

I lost my first 100 pounds and I felt so light I wanted to dance. But I started to gain it back, and I realized I had to go deeper and deal with the root of my problem—the unfelt pain. I began therapy, joined a Twelve-Step program and accepted the love and support of my family and friends. At 35, I cried for the first time since I was eight. Feeling my pain was the true secret of my weight loss.

Once I turned that corner, it was up to me to continue the work and to be conscious one day at a time. It was a process of growing self-knowledge and self-acceptance. I continued my therapy. I started to study nutrition, and I learned that for me, eating fat is a sedative. I watched my behavior and monitored what brought on my need to eat. When I found myself knee-deep in Häagen-Dazs, I stopped and asked myself how I got there.

Though there were times when I would backslide, it was my acceptance of myself in all my strengths *and* weaknesses that helped me get back up and keep going. My goal was to be better—not perfect.

When I see childhood obesity now, it breaks my heart. We wouldn't dream of laughing at a child who has no arm or leg or who uses a wheelchair. But people will tease and ostracize a child who has an eating disorder and is obese. We still don't understand that the weight such a child carries is the weight of that child's own pain.

Healing my life wasn't just about losing weight. I had to learn how to live life as an adult. I had never learned basic social skills—once, at work, a man talked to me at the water cooler and I giggled like a 14-year-old girl. I started the process of learning about relationships and growing up.

Now, at 46, I am an adult. I have become a person I truly love. My weight is in the average range, I exercise regularly and I have a career I love as a motivational speaker. I recognize the good things that came from my years of childhood pain and isolation: my love for classical music, my ability to sew and to do stained glass—to create beauty with my hands. Even my ability to speak well and engagingly can be traced to the many hours I spent watching such great entertainers as Lucille Ball and Milton Berle on TV.

I am grateful for the blessings in my life now, and I accept the events in my life as gifts of growth that create strength of character and strength of faith. Today I cry in gratitude for the life I have.

Joan Fountain with Carol Kline

4

ON MARRIAGE

Now you will feel no rain,
For each of you will be shelter to the other.
Now you will feel no cold,
For each of you will be warmth to the other.
Now there is no more loneliness for you,
For each of you will be companion to the
other.
Now you are two bodies,
But there is only one life before you.
Go now to your dwelling place,
To enter into the days of your togetherness.
And may your days be good, and long upon
the earth.

Apache blessing

Home Forever

The most precious possession that ever comes to a man in this world is a woman's heart.

Josiah G. Holland

It was one of those rare days. You know the kind I mean. When I woke up in the morning, I felt at peace with the world. The sun was shining. The air was crisp with the smell of green. It was a beautiful day and all was well with the world.

It was my day off and I actually looked forward to doing the housecleaning and laundry. I work at a very busy long-term care facility as a rehabilitation nurse, and some days I welcome the kind of diversion that housework offers. Not always. But at times it is a refreshing change.

The phone rang around 8:00 A.M. On the other end of the line I could hear my mother's voice. It was somewhat strained, and instinctively I knew something was wrong. She was on the verge of tears.

She proceeded to tell me that my grandfather, her father, was terribly upset because the nursing home he had been admitted to two weeks earlier still had not placed him in a room with my grandmother. That had been the deal: he was to share a room with his wife. We had promised him that, and he had counted on it.

Seven-and-a-half years earlier, Grandma had been placed in a nursing home due to progressing Alzheimer's and my grandfather's inability to care for her. She was 90 at the time of her admission, and he was 91. Every day for the next seven-and-a-half years, he walked a mile each way to spend his days with her. He fed her her meals, combed her hair, stroked her, spoke softly to her and told her how much he loved her. Although she was unable to speak or return his care and compassion, Grandpa continued his daily vigil.

Every time I visited, he told me the story of the day they first met—a day he said he would never forget. He told me how he first saw her through a crowd of people at the fair, and how he was struck by the "lovely red bow she wore in her beautiful brown hair." He then would take out his wallet and show me the picture of her from that day at the fair. He carried it with him always. I remember him showing it to me as a small child.

Eventually, Grandpa also became too frail to live alone and care for himself. At times, he was even forgetting to eat. We knew it was only a matter of time before he, too, would have to be cared for by others.

This was not an easy thing for him to accept. He was a man who had always been fiercely independent. He owned and drove a car until he was 93, and he golfed daily, when the weather permitted, until he was 96. He paid his own bills, maintained his apartment, washed his own clothes and shopped for and cooked his own meals until he was 97. But at almost 98 years of age, he could no longer care for himself.

With a lot of coaxing, love and support, Grandpa agreed to be admitted to the nursing home my grandmother was in. But only on one condition: He would share a room with my grandmother or he wouldn't go. That was his stipulation and the family agreed. He wanted, as he said, "to be with his sweetheart."

The director of nursing at the facility agreed to the request and Grandpa was admitted to the nursing home. Upon admission, however, she stated that it would be a day or two until they could move my grandmother's roommate out and put Grandpa into her room. We assured Grandpa that all was well. We left, assuming everything was taken care of.

But the days passed into weeks, and Grandpa still had not moved in with my grandmother. He was becoming increasingly confused and lethargic. He did not understand why he couldn't be with her. Worse, he was on a different floor and couldn't even "find" her.

Although my mother kept asking why Grandpa hadn't been moved and what the delay was all about, her questions fell on deaf ears. Finally, she was told by the director of nursing that they felt it would not be in Grandpa's best interest to move him in with my grandmother. They seemed to feel that in his frail condition, he might hurt himself trying to care for her. They had, after all, watched him dote over her for over seven years. They felt he might hurt himself trying to reposition or move her. They knew him well. They knew his independent nature—his will to do things right.

At first, my mother accepted their decision, but later she became increasingly concerned. Grandpa was not faring well separated from his wife. He wanted only to be with her—his "sweetheart " of 68 years. He talked about it constantly. And he was always sad. The twinkle in his beautiful blue eyes was fading.

On the morning my phone rang, I had not seen Grandpa since his admission. As my mother, fighting back her tears, told me what had happened, a genuine sadness came over me. The grandfather I loved so dearly, that I had idolized as a child and grown to know and respect as an adult, was spending his final years disheartened and lonely. He, my tie with infinity, was losing his spirit. He was being denied choices and control over his life. I became incensed at what I felt was truly an injustice.

After talking to my mother, I decided to take matters into my own hands. I called the director of nursing at the facility and inquired about the situation. She reiterated the information my mother had given me. I calmly explained that I felt that Grandpa should be moved into a room with my grandmother, as promised. She continued to insist that he might overdo it and hurt himself in caring for Grandma. I insisted that it was important that the promise be kept, and said that they would both benefit emotionally from the shared room. After all, they had shared a room for 68 years. I saw no reason why, at the end of their long and loving lives, they should be denied each other's companionship. They loved each other dearly and being together had been the "deal."

After much discussion and disagreement, I could not contain myself any longer. My emotions went wild. I asked, "What's the point? If my grandfather, who is 98 years old, had high cholesterol and absolutely loved to eat cheese—guess what? I'd let him. As a matter of fact, I'd go out and buy all his favorite cheeses for him! And if he couldn't feed himself, I would. Being in a room with my grandmother is important to him. Important to his emotional well-being. Important to his spirit. Important for the twinkle in his eyes."

There was a long pause on the other end of the phone. I was then told by the director of nursing that she understood what I was saying and would take care of it.

It was about 9:00 A.M. when I finished speaking with the director of nursing, and I told her that she had until 2:00 P.M. that afternoon to move my grandparents into a room together. I also informed her that if the transfer was not done by that time, then I would personally remove them both from the facility and place them elsewhere—where they could share a room.

I then called my mother and said, "Drop everything and get your purse. We're going to see Grandma and Grandpa." I drove to my mom's, stopping on the way to buy a color TV for Grandpa. Mom met me at the door with a smile on her face, and together we drove to the nursing home, feeling wonderfully in control of the situation.

When we arrived, Grandma was sleeping soundly and Grandpa was sitting next to her, stroking her hair. He had a smile on his face and that old familiar twinkle in his wonderful blue eyes. He fussed with her covers, straightening the linens on her bed. And he began to tell me once again about his "sweetheart" and how much he loved her. He chattered on about the fair and the red bow in her beautiful brown hair. He showed me the picture in his wallet. He was finally home.

Jean Bole

A Little Holiday Magic

Christmas Eve has always been my favorite day of the year. December 24, 1969, I was on my own, living in my first apartment. With several hours to fill before joining my family at Mother's, I decided to do a little last-minute shopping.

On the third floor of our city's oldest and finest department store, I bought a large basket of gourmet cheeses, smoked oysters, a bottle of wine and wineglasses to take to my family. On my way down, the elevator stopped at the second floor, where everyone but an older couple and me got off—and where a tall, handsome man in a navy suit got on. We started down again; then suddenly, there was a loud thud. The elevator jerked, then stalled. We were stuck—on Christmas Eve!

Luckily the elevator was equipped with a phone, and the older man called someone in maintenance, who assured us we would soon be moving again. Thirty minutes passed while we made small talk, then placed another call. We learned that the elevator needed a new part and we were in for a long wait.

At that point, one by one, we—the older couple, Mr.

and Mrs. Phillips; John, the handsome man in navy; and I—sat down on the floor and began sharing Christmas memories. An hour passed, then two; we found ourselves so involved in the conversation that we forgot we were trapped. As we took turns revealing bits and pieces of our pasts, we shared my basket of cheese and wine. I didn't realize it at the time, but what we were doing was creating another special Christmas memory.

After five hours, the elevator finally moved. When the doors opened, the worried store manager, relieved to find us in such good spirits, handed out gift baskets of gourmet cheese. Saying our good-byes, the four of us exchanged addresses and promised to send holiday greetings to each other in the years to come.

I got to my mother's for our traditional family Christmas—a bit late, but I got there. As I closed my eyes that night, I saw not visions of sugarplums, but a handsome man in a navy suit.

Christmas evening I returned to my apartment loaded down with gifts. Waiting for me was a single red rose and an envelope slipped under the door. Inside the envelope was a message: *I could really use some help with this cheese basket. John.* At the bottom was his phone number . . .

John and I were married the following Christmas Eve in a sunset ceremony on a Hawaiian beach. That was many years ago, and we are still exchanging Christmas greetings with Mr. and Mrs. Phillips and enjoying a basket of gourmet cheese and wine for our midnight snack every Christmas Eve. And I still wake up every Christmas Eve morning filled with excitement at the magic of the day.

K. M. Jenkins

Paris in the Springtime

I was in the garden tending my roses one spring day when Dan got down on his knees and asked me to marry him. I told him to ask me again in three months. After all, we had had our ups and downs, and I wasn't sure either of us was ready for that type of commitment.

Three months came and went. He didn't ask again, and we cautiously went on as before, practicing with renewed commitment the fine art of relationship.

That winter we began planning a spring trip to Paris. I didn't quite know why, but my heart and soul were crying for Paris, and I'd always had a strong desire to experience that city with Dan. Now that desire was being fulfilled.

Paris was incredible! Having been fluent in French 20 years earlier, I quickly became Dan's translator. My French was a disaster, but since Dan hardly spoke a word of it, he thought it was perfect. He never tired of hearing me trying to apologize to waiters for slaughtering their exquisite language, or attempting to order something I'd be able to recognize when it arrived at the table.

Romance was in the air everywhere we went, and Dan was constantly asking me how to say things in French like "kiss" and "give me your hand" and "I love you." We boated on the Seine, walked along tree-lined boulevards for hours, drank coffee at sidewalk cafés, and fell deeply in love all over again.

One evening, after we had just been seated in a small, quaint restaurant, Dan leaned toward me and asked, "How do you say 'Will you marry me?' in French?" I told him I wasn't sure, but I thought it would be, *Veux-tu me marier?*

Veux-tu me marier? he repeated.

"Honey, that's great!" I said. "Your pronunciation is really getting good!"

"No," he said emphatically. *Veux-tu me marier?* And he pushed a small velvet box across the table.

I opened the box and saw two beautiful rings—an engagement and a wedding ring—and it dawned on me what was happening. As tears rolled down my face, all the waiters came rushing over to stand around the table, fussing over us and exclaiming how wonderful it was. They were still taking photographs of us when I looked at Dan and finally said, *"Oui, chéri!"*

Jennifer Read Hawthorne

Marriage Advice from 1886

Let your love be stronger than your hate or anger.
Learn the wisdom of compromise, for it is better to bend
a little than to break.
Believe the best rather than the worst.
People have a way of living up or down to your opinion
of them.
Remember that true friendship is the basis for any lasting
relationship. The person you choose to marry is deserv-
ing of the courtesies and kindnesses you bestow on
your friends.
Please hand this down to your children and your children's children: The more things change the more they
are the same.

Jane Wells (1886)
Submitted by Carol Abbs

A Handful of Emeralds

Life isn't a matter of milestones, but of moments.

Rose Kennedy

When Jeff and I got married 16 years ago on a blustery Saturday, it never crossed our minds that the day would come when it would seem like a long time ago. Since that time, we've lived in eight towns and had three children. We're on our third bottle of Tabasco sauce and I just tore up the last of the sheets we got as wedding gifts for cleaning rags. Unfortunately, most of the horrible earth-tone furniture we bought for our first apartment survives. My wedding dress hangs in the back of my closet. I can still zip it up (as long as I'm not in it). We've gone through four cars (alas—none of them new), and too many ups and downs to count.

One day stands out in my memory. We were living out East and my folks had come to visit. Because we were broke and exhausted new parents, Mom and Dad kindly footed the bill for a week in a beach house at the Jersey shore. The arrangement was hard on Jeff's ego, I was in a foul mood myself, and he and I had an enormously stupid quarrel over a game of Monopoly. He stalked out of the house and across the street to the beach. A couple of hours later, as I waited for him on the shore, he emerged from the Atlantic badly sunburned, carrying an air mattress.

"Where's your wedding ring?" I demanded.

He looked down at his left hand, stricken. His finger had constricted from the cold water as he drifted on the raft. The ring slipped off and was out there with the sea anemones. I started to cry.

"Take your ring off and throw it out in the ocean, too," he begged me.

"Why on earth would I throw away gold when we don't have enough money to buy gas to get home?" I wailed.

"Because both of our rings would be out in the ocean together."

Practicality won out over hearts and flowers, and I wear my ring to this day. That memory, however, has kept me going through many a time that was far from romantic.

When our anniversary rolls around, I think of that day on the beach. And I think of what the late Charlie MacArthur told Helen Hayes when he met her at a party. He gave her a handful of peanuts and said, "I wish these were emeralds."

After they had been happily married for many years and MacArthur was near the end of his life, he gave her a handful of emeralds and said, "I wish these were peanuts."

Me, too.

Rebecca Christian

What Women Don't Understand About Guys

Contrary to what many women believe, it's easy to develop a long-term, intimate and mutually fulfilling relationship with a guy. Of course, the guy has to be a Labrador retriever. With human guys, it's extremely difficult. This is because guys don't really grasp what women mean by the word *relationship*.

Let's say a guy named Roger asks a woman named Elaine out to a movie. She accepts; they have a pretty good time. A few nights later he asks her out to dinner, and again they enjoy themselves. They continue to see each other regularly, and soon neither is seeing anybody else.

Then one evening when they're driving home, a thought occurs to Elaine. She says: "Do you realize that we've been seeing each other for exactly six months?"

Silence fills the car. To Elaine, it seems like a very loud silence. She thinks to herself: "Geez, I wonder if it bothers him that I said that. Maybe he feels confined by our relationship. Maybe he thinks I'm trying to push him into some kind of obligation."

And Roger is thinking: "Gosh. Six months."

And Elaine is thinking: "But hey, *I'm* not so sure I want this kind of relationship either. Are we heading toward marriage? Toward children? Toward a *lifetime* together? Am I ready for that level of commitment? Do I really even *know* this person?"

And Roger is thinking: "So that means it was . . . let's see . . . February when we started going out, which was right after I had the car at the dealer's, which means . . . lemme check the odometer . . . whoa! I am *way* overdue for an oil change here."

And Elaine is thinking: "He's upset. I can see it on his face. Maybe I'm reading this completely wrong. Maybe he wants *more* from our relationship—more intimacy, more commitment. Maybe he senses my reservations. Yes, that's it. He's afraid of being rejected."

And Roger is thinking: "I'm going to have them look at the transmission again. I don't care what those morons say—it's still not shifting right. And they better not try to blame it on cold weather this time. It's 87 degrees out, and this thing is shifting like a garbage truck, and I paid those incompetent, thieving cretins *600 dollars!*"

And Elaine is thinking: "He's angry, and I don't blame him. I'd be angry too. I feel so guilty, putting him through this, but I can't help the way I feel. I'm just not sure."

And Roger is thinking: "They'll probably say it's only a 90-day warranty. That's what they're gonna say!"

And Elaine is thinking: "Maybe I'm too idealistic, waiting for a knight to come riding up on his white horse, when I'm sitting next to a perfectly good person who's in pain because of my self-centered, schoolgirl fantasy."

And Roger is thinking: "Warranty? I'll give them a warranty!"

"Roger," Elaine says aloud.

"What?" says Roger.

"I'm such a fool," Elaine says, sobbing. "I mean, I know there's no knight and there's no horse."

"There's no horse?" says Roger.

"You think I'm a fool, don't you?" Elaine says.

"No!" Roger says, glad to know the correct answer.

"It's just that . . . I need some time," Elaine says.

There is a 15-second pause while Roger tries to come up with a safe response. "Yes," he finally says.

Elaine, deeply moved, touches his hand. "Oh, Roger, do you really feel that way?"

"What way?" says Roger.

"That way about time," Elaine says.

"Oh," says Roger. "Yes."

Elaine gazes deeply into his eyes, causing him to become very nervous about what she might say next, especially if it involves a horse. At last she says, "Thank you, Roger."

"Thank *you*," he responds.

Then he takes her home, and she lies on her bed, a conflicted soul weeping until dawn, whereas when Roger gets back to his place, he opens a bag of chips, turns on the TV and immediately becomes deeply involved in a rerun of a tennis match between two Czech players he never heard of. A tiny voice in his mind tells him that something major was going on back there in the car, but he figures it's better not to think about it.

The next day Elaine will call her closest friend, and they will talk for six straight hours. In painstaking detail they will analyze everything she said and everything he said. They will continue to discuss this subject for weeks, never reaching any definite conclusions but never getting bored with it either.

Meanwhile, Roger, playing racquetball one day with a friend of his and Elaine's, will pause just before serving and ask, "Norm, did Elaine ever own a horse?"

We're not talking about different wavelengths here. We're talking about different *planets* in completely different *solar systems*. Elaine cannot communicate meaningfully with Roger because the sum total of his thinking about relationships is *Huh?*

He has a guy brain, basically an analytical, problem-solving organ. It's not comfortable with nebulous concepts such as love, need and trust. If the guy brain has to form an opinion about another person, it prefers to base it on facts, such as his or her earned-run average.

Women have trouble accepting this. They are convinced that guys *must* spend a certain amount of time thinking about the relationship. How could a guy see another human being day after day, night after night, and *not* be thinking about the relationship? This is what women figure.

They are wrong. A guy in a relationship is like an ant standing on top of a truck tire. The ant is aware that something large is there, but he cannot even dimly comprehend what it is. And if the truck starts moving and the tire starts to roll, the ant will sense that something important is happening, but right up until he rolls around to the bottom and is squashed, the only thought in his tiny brain will be *Huh?*

Thus the No. 1 tip for women to remember is never assume the guy understands that you and he have a relationship. You have to plant the idea in his brain by constantly making subtle references to it, such as:

"Roger, would you mind passing me the sugar, inasmuch as we have a relationship?"

"Wake up, Roger! There's a prowler in the den and we have a relationship! You and I do, I mean."

"Good news, Roger! The doctor says we're going to have our fourth child—another indication that we have a relationship!"

"Roger, inasmuch as this plane is crashing and we have only a minute to live, I want you to know that we've had a wonderful 53 years of marriage together, which clearly constitutes a relationship."

Never let up, women. Pound away relentlessly at this concept, and eventually it will start to penetrate the guy's brain. Someday he might even start thinking about it on his own. He'll be talking with some other guys about women, and out of the blue he'll say, "Elaine and I, we have, ummm . . . we have, ahhh . . . we . . . we have this thing."

And he will sincerely mean it.

Dave Barry

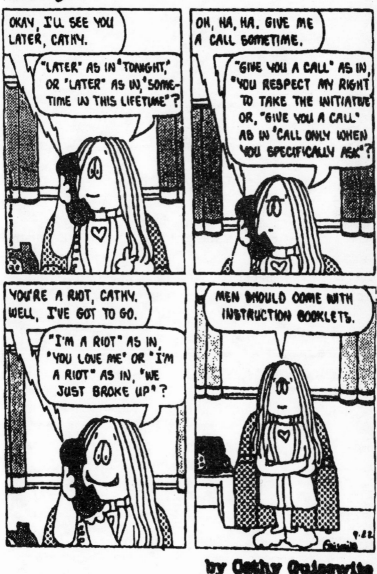

©Cathy. Distributed by Universal Press Syndicate. Reprinted with permission. All rights reserved.

Lost and Found

Winona was 19 when she first met Edward, a tall, handsome young man, in the summer of 1928. He had come to Detroit to visit his sister, who was engaged to Winona's brother. Edward stayed with some friends, and although he was there for only a few days, there was enough time to get to know the lively, dark-haired young woman who intrigued him from their first meeting. They promised to write, and Edward returned to Pittsburgh.

For many months, they wrote long, newsy letters sharing details of their lives and their dreams. Then as quickly as he came into her life, Edward left. His letters stopped, and Winona gradually accepted that he simply wasn't interested anymore. Edward couldn't understand why Winona had stopped writing, and he, too, resigned himself to the fact that the woman he had fallen in love with did not return his love.

Several years later, Winona married Robert, a dashing man 10 years her senior. They had three sons. She got news of Ed's life through her sister-in-law. Several years after Winona married, Edward got married, and he, too, had three children.

On one of her visits to her brother and sister-in-law's in Buffalo, her brother announced, "We're driving to Pittsburgh to Ed's daughter's wedding. Do you want to come?" Winona didn't hesitate, and off they went.

She was nervous in the car just thinking about what she would say to this man she hadn't seen in 30 years. Would he remember their letters? Would he have time to talk with her? Would he even want to?

Soon after they got to the wedding reception, Ed spotted Winona from the other side of the room. He walked slowly over to her. Winona's heart was racing as they shook hands and said hello. When they sat at one of the long tables to talk, Winona's heart was beating so hard she was afraid that Ed could hear it. Edward had tears in his eyes as they exchanged polite conversation about the wedding and their respective families. They never mentioned the letters, and after a few minutes, Ed returned to his duties as father of the bride.

Winona returned to Detroit, where she continued teaching piano lessons, working at an advertising agency, and, as always, making the best of whatever life offered. She tucked away the memory of her brief visit with Ed along with her other memories of him.

When Ed's wife died 10 years later, Winona sent him a sympathy card. Two years after that, Winona's husband died and Ed wrote to her. Once again, they were corresponding.

Ed wrote often, and his letters became the highlight of Winona's day. On her way to work, she stopped by the post office to pick up his letters, and then she read them at the stoplights. By the end of her half-hour drive, the letters were read and Winona had a happy start to her day. Gradually, Edward expressed his love for his "darling Winona," and they arranged for him to come to Detroit for his vacation.

Winona was excited and nervous about the visit. After all, except for their brief meeting at the wedding, they hadn't spent any time together in over 40 years. They had only been writing for six months, and Edward was coming for two weeks.

It was a lovely, warm June day when Winona drove to the airport to pick up Edward. This time when he saw Winona, he rushed to her and wrapped her in a long, loving hug. They chatted happily and comfortably as they retrieved luggage and found their way to the car. It was an easy beginning.

When they were in the car on their way to Edward's hotel, he pulled a small velvet box out of his pocket and slipped an engagement ring on Winona's finger. She was speechless. He had hinted at marriage in his letters, but this was too sudden and too soon. Or was it? Hadn't she waited all these years to know this love?

For two weeks, Ed wooed his Winona. He even wrote her letters from his hotel. Winona's concerns gradually dissolved in the stream of Ed's love and the whole-hearted support of her family and friends. On September 18, 1971, dressed in a long pink gown, Winona was escorted down the aisle on the arm of her oldest son. She and Ed were married and in Winona's words, "We lived happily ever after."

And those letters that had suddenly stopped so many years before? It turns out that Edward's mother had destroyed Winona's letters because she didn't want to lose her youngest son. Forty-three years later, Winona found him.

Elinor Daily Hall

Grandpa's Valentine

I was the only family member living close by, so I
received the initial call from the nursing home. Grandpa
was failing rapidly. I should come. There was nothing to
do but hold his hand. "I love you, Grandpa. Thank you for
always being there for me." And silently, I released him.

Memories . . . memories . . . six days a week, the farmer
in the old blue shirt and bib overalls caring for those
Hereford cattle he loved so much . . . on hot summer days
lifting bales of hay from the wagon, plowing the soil,
planting the corn and beans and harvesting them in the
fall . . . always working from dawn to dusk. Survival
demanded the work, work, work.

But on Sundays, after the morning chores were done, he
put on his gray suit and hat. Grandma wore her wine-
colored dress and the ivory beads, and they went to church.
There was little other social life. Grandpa and Grandma
were quiet, peaceful, unemotional people who every day
did what they had to do. He was my grandpa—he had been
for 35 years. It was hard to picture him in any other role.

The nurse apologized for having to ask me so soon to
please remove Grandpa's things from the room. It would

not take long. There wasn't much. Then I found *it* in the top drawer of his nightstand. It looked like a very old handmade valentine. What must have been red paper at one time was a streaked faded pink. A piece of white paper had been glued to the center of the heart. On it, penned in Grandma's handwriting, were these words:

> *TO LEE FROM HARRIET*
> *With All My Love,*
> *February 14, 1895*

> *Are you alive? Real? Or are you the most beautiful dream that I have had in years? Are you an angel—or a figment of my imagination? Someone I fabricated to fill the void? To soothe the pain? Where did you find the time to listen? How could you understand?*
>
> *You made me laugh when my heart was crying. You took me dancing when I couldn't take a step. You helped me set new goals when I was dying. You showed me dew drops and I had diamonds. You brought me wildflowers and I had orchids. You sang to me and angelic choirs burst forth in song. You held my hand and my whole being loved you. You gave me a ring and I belonged to you. I belonged to you and I have experienced all.*

Tears streamed down my cheeks as I read the words. I pictured the old couple I had always known. It's difficult to imagine your grandparents in any role other than that. What I read was so very beautiful and sacred. Grandpa had kept it all those years. Now it is framed on my dresser, a treasured part of family history.

Elaine Reese

A Soldier's Last Letter

A week before the Battle of Bull Run (also known as Manassas), Sullivan Ballou, a major in the 2nd Rhode Island Volunteers, wrote home to his wife in Smithfield:

July 14, 1861
Washington, D. C.

My very dear Sarah,

The indications are very strong that we shall move in a few days, perhaps tomorrow. Lest I should not be able to write you again, I feel impelled to write a few lines that may fall under your eye when I shall be no more.

I have no misgivings about or lack of confidence in the cause in which I am engaged, and my courage does not halt or falter. I know how strongly American civilization now leans on the triumph of the government, and how great a debt we owe to those who went before us through the blood and suffering of the Revolution. And I am willing—perfectly willing—to lay down all my joys in this life to help maintain this government and to pay that debt.

Sarah, my love for you is deathless. It seems to bind me with mighty cables that nothing but Omnipotence could break. And yet my love of country comes over me like a strong wind and bears me irresistibly, with all these chains, to the battlefield.

The memory of all the blissful moments I have enjoyed with you come crowding over me, and I feel most deeply grateful to God and you that I have enjoyed them so long. And how hard it is for me to give them up and burn to ashes the hopes of future years when, God willing, we might still have lived and loved together and seen our sons grow up to honorable manhood around us. . . .

If I do not return, my dear Sarah, never forget how much I love you, nor that when my last breath escapes me on the battlefield, it will whisper your name. Forgive my many faults and the many pains I have caused you. How thoughtless, how foolish I have sometimes been.

But, oh Sarah! If the dead can come back to this earth and flit unseen around those they love, I shall always be with you in the brightest days and in the darkest nights. Always. Always.

And when the soft breeze fans your cheek, it shall be my breath; and as the cool air fans your throbbing temple, it shall be my spirit passing by. Sarah, do not mourn me dead: Think I am gone and wait for me, for we shall meet again.

Maj. Sullivan Ballou
Submitted by Nancy Wong

EDITORS' NOTE: Sullivan Ballou was killed a week later at the first Battle of Bull Run.

A Love Like That

Nobody has ever measured, not even poets, how much the heart can hold.

Zelda Fitzgerald

I was 23, and all the way to the hospital I'd been composing what I would say to Mama before they took her to cut into her heart, whose center I supposed myself to be; hadn't she told me all my life I was the most important thing in the world to her?

Threading my way through the hospital corridors, I practiced my opening line, which had to strike just the right note. Who but I could give her the strength and confidence she would need? Whose face but mine would she want to be the last one she saw before they cut her open and she died probably? Whose kiss but mine . . .?

I turned a corner and there was my mother lying on a stretcher in the hall, waiting for them to come for her. My father was standing over her. Something about the two of them made me stop and then, as I watched, made me keep my distance, as if there were a wall between us, and around them.

It was clear to me at that moment that for them, nothing existed outside them, nothing; there was only the man, the woman. She didn't see me, nor from the looks of it care much whether she did. They weren't talking. He was holding her hand. She was smiling into his eyes; and they were, I swear, speaking a language that at 23 I hadn't begun to understand, much less speak myself. But I could see them do it, literally see them, and I moved closer to see more, stunned, fascinated, very jealous that I had fallen in love with someone, married him, divorced him and never once come close to what I was looking at in that hall.

Next time, I said, I will know better. I will love like that.

Linda Ellerbee

All the Days of My Life

My mother and father were about to celebrate their 50th anniversary. Mother called, all excited. "He got me a dozen white roses!" Sounding like a teenager who'd just been asked to the prom, she talked about how happy she was, how good she felt and how lucky she was.

This anniversary brought out a side of my parents that I never knew. For instance, their wedding rings are each inscribed with a line of poetry: *I send you a cream-white rosebud.* My father told me this in the kitchen one day. My mother said, "Oh, John," as if to stop him. My father said, "Oh, Claire."

That's the way my parents have always been about their relationship: private. There was never any mushy stuff going on that we kids could see. What we did see was buddies, a team.

"Do you remember the poem?" I asked my dad that day in the kitchen, as I examined his wedding ring under the light. He looked at me, took a breath and started reciting "A White Rose" by the Irish-American poet John Boyle O'Reilly. He didn't stumble once; it was as if he had been reciting it in his head every day for the last half-century.

"The red rose whispers of passion, / And the white rose breathes of love," he began.

My mother said, "Oh, John!"

"O, the red rose is a falcon, / And the white rose is a dove."

"Oh, John!" My mother said. Then she left the room.

"But I send you a cream-white rosebud / With a flush on its petal tips," he went on, standing there by the sink. *"For the love that is purest and sweetest / Has a kiss of desire on the lips."*

My father stopped. "Isn't that beautiful?" he said, smiling.

We went to find my mother, who was in the den, her head in her hands. "It's beautiful!" I said to her.

"It's embarrassing," she said.

This is a woman who in her youth had never seen a happy marriage and wondered why anyone would bother. Instead, she imagined a future as a Chaucer scholar. In college she found dating only mildly amusing. But then she met my father.

He was the most fundamentally decent man she had ever met. It was the man, not the institution of marriage, that drew her. She went to the altar, she later told us, feeling as if she were jumping off a cliff.

In their first year of marriage, my father went off to war. My mother was five months pregnant, and terrified. She had the baby and waited. She ate chocolate-nut sundaes to soothe her heart.

My father returned, said hello to his seven-month-old son and, with my mother, soon bought a house. Then they had a daughter, then another daughter and then me.

Even as a kid, I could tell my parents were different. Dad preferred being with Mom to going off bowling with the guys. And when he wasn't around, she didn't roll her eyes and make jokes at her husband's expense as other wives did. Instead, she'd say, "You know, he's never disappointed me."

To celebrate their 50th anniversary, my parents renewed their wedding vows in church. Some 75 friends were watching. When my father repeated his vows, he choked up and had to pause. My mother said hers with more passion than I'd ever heard her use. Staring into his eyes, she proclaimed, ". . . all the days of my life."

After the ceremony we had a big party, where my father kissed my mother and said, "Welcome to eternity."

She was speechless much of the time, except when she declared, "This is the happiest day of my life." Then she added, "This is better than my wedding day—because now I know how it all works out!"

Jeanne Marie Laskas

5

ON
MOTHERHOOD

Making the decision to have a child—it's momentous. It is to decide forever to have your heart go walking around outside your body.

Elizabeth Stone

It Will Change Your Life

Time is running out for my friend. We are sitting at lunch when she casually mentions that she and her husband are thinking of "starting a family." What she means is that her biological clock has begun its countdown, and she is being forced to consider the prospect of motherhood.

"We're taking a survey," she says, half joking. "Do you think I should have a baby?"

"It will change your life," I say carefully, keeping my tone neutral.

"I know," she says. "No more sleeping in on Saturdays, no more spontaneous vacations . . ."

But that is not what I mean at all. I look at my friend, trying to decide what to tell her.

I want her to know what she will never learn in childbirth classes. I want to tell her that the physical wounds of childbearing heal, but that becoming a mother will leave her with an emotional wound so raw that she will be forever vulnerable.

I consider warning her that she will never read a newspaper again without asking, "What if that had been my child?" That every plane crash, every fire will haunt her. That when she sees pictures of starving children, she will wonder if anything could be worse than watching your child die.

I look at her carefully manicured nails and stylish suit and think that no matter how sophisticated she is, becoming a mother will reduce her to the primitive level of a bear protecting her cub. That an urgent call of "Mom!" will cause her to drop a soufflé or her best crystal without a moment's hesitation.

I feel I should warn her that no matter how many years she has invested in her career, she will be professionally derailed by motherhood. She might arrange for child care, but one day she will be going into an important business meeting and she will think about her baby's sweet smell. She will have to use every ounce of discipline to keep from running home, just to make sure her child is all right.

I want my friend to know that everyday decisions will no longer be routine. That a five-year-old boy's desire to go to the men's room rather than the women's at McDonald's will become a major dilemma. That right there, in the midst of clattering trays and screaming children, issues of independence and gender identity will be weighed against the prospect that a child molester may be lurking in the restroom. However decisive she may be at the office, she will second-guess herself constantly as a mother.

Looking at my attractive friend, I want to assure her that eventually she will shed the pounds of pregnancy, but she will never feel the same about herself. That her life, now so important, will be of less value to her once she has a child. That she would give it up in a moment to save her offspring, but will also begin to hope for more years— not to accomplish her own dreams, but to watch her child accomplish his. I want her to know that a cesarean scar or shiny stretch marks will become badges of honor.

My friend's relationship with her husband will change, but not in the ways she thinks. I wish she could understand how much more you can love a man who is always careful to powder the baby or who never hesitates to play with his son or daughter. I think she should know that she will fall in love with her husband again for reasons she would now find very unromantic.

I wish my friend could sense the bond she will feel with women throughout history who have tried desperately to stop war and prejudice and drunk driving. I hope she will understand why I can think rationally about most issues, but become temporarily insane when I discuss the threat of nuclear war to my children's future.

I want to describe to my friend the exhilaration of seeing your child learn to hit a baseball. I want to capture for her the belly laugh of a baby who is touching the soft fur of a dog for the first time. I want her to taste the joy that is so real it hurts.

My friend's quizzical look makes me realize that tears have formed in my eyes. "You'll never regret it," I say finally. Then I reach across the table, squeeze my friend's hand, and offer a prayer for her and me and all of the mere mortal women who stumble their way into this holiest of callings.

Dale Hanson Bourke
Submitted by Karen Wheeler

As I Watch You Sleep

My precious child, I have slipped into your room to sit with you as you sleep, and watch the rise and fall of your breath for a while. Your eyes are peacefully closed, and your soft blond curls frame your cherubic face. Just moments ago, as I sat with my paperwork in the den, a mounting sadness came over me, while I contemplated the day's events. I could no longer keep my attention on my work, and so I have come to talk to you in the silence, as you rest.

In the morning, I was impatient with you as you dawdled and dressed slowly, telling you to stop being such a slow-poke. I scolded you for misplacing your lunch ticket, and I capped off breakfast with a disapproving look as you spilt food on your shirt. "Again?" I sighed and shook my head. You just smiled sheepishly at me and said, "Bye, Mommy!"

In the afternoon, I made phone calls while you played in your room, singing aloud and gesturing to yourself, with all of your toys lined up in jovial rows on the bed. I motioned irritably for you to be quiet and stop all the racket, and then proceeded to spend another busy hour on the phone. "Get your homework done right now," I later rattled off like a sergeant, "and stop wasting so much time." "Okay, Mom," you said remorsefully, sitting up straight at your desk with pencil in hand. After that, it was quiet in your room.

In the evening, as I worked at my desk, you approached me hesitantly. "Will we read a story tonight, Mom?" you asked with a glimmer of hope. "Not tonight," I said abruptly, "your room is still a mess! How many times will I have to remind you?" You wandered off in a shuffle with your head down and headed for your room. Before long, you were back, peering around the edge of the door. "Now what do you want?" I asked in an agitated tone of voice.

You didn't say a word, you just came bounding in the room, threw your arms around my neck and kissed me on the cheek. "Good night, Mommy, I love you," was all you said, as you squeezed tightly. And then, as swiftly as you had appeared, you were gone.

After that, I sat with my eyes fixed on my desk for a long time, feeling a wave of remorse come over me. At what point did I lose the rhythm of the day, I wondered, and at what cost? You hadn't done anything to evoke my mood. You were just being a child, busy about the task of growing and learning. I got lost today, in an adult world of responsibilities and demands, and had little energy left to give to you. You became my teacher today, with your unrestrained urge to rush in and kiss me good-night, even after an arduous day of tip-toeing around my moods.

And now, as I see you lying fast asleep, I yearn for the day to start all over again. Tomorrow, I will treat myself with as much understanding as you have shown me today, so that I can be a real mom—offering a warm smile when you awaken, a word of encouragement after school, and an animated story before bed. I will laugh when you laugh and cry when you cry. I will remind myself that you are a child, not a grownup, and I will enjoy being your mom. Your resilient spirit has touched me today, and so, I come to you in this late hour to thank you, my child, my teacher and my friend, for the gift of your love.

Diane Loomans

To My Grown-Up Son

My hands were busy through the day
I didn't have much time to play
The little games you asked me to,
I didn't have much time for you.
I'd wash your clothes, I'd sew and cook,
But when you'd bring your picture book
And asked me please to share your fun,
I'd say, "A little later, Son."
I'd tuck you in all safe at night
And hear your prayers, turn out the light,
Then tiptoe softly to the door . . .
I wish I'd stayed a minute more.

For life is short, the years rush past . . .
A little boy grows up so fast.
No longer is he at your side,
His precious secrets to confide.
The picture books are put away,
There are no longer games to play,
No good-night kiss, no prayers to hear,
That all belongs to yesteryear.

My hands, once busy, now are still.
The days are long and hard to fill.
I wish I could go back and do
The little things you asked me to!

Author Unknown
Submitted by Eleanor Newbern

Running Away

On a very hectic day when my husband and I were busy going in a hundred directions, our four-and-a-half-year-old son, Justin Carl, had to be reprimanded for getting into mischief. After several attempts, my husband George finally told him to stand in the corner. He was very quiet but wasn't too happy about it. Finally, after a few moments, he said, "I'm going to run away from home."

My first reaction was surprise, and his words angered me. "You are?" I blurted. But as I turned to look at him, he looked like an angel, so small, so innocent, with his face so sad.

As my heart felt his pain, I remembered a moment in my own childhood when I spoke those words and how unloved and lonely I felt. He was saying so much more than just his words. He was crying from within, "Don't you dare ignore me. Please notice me! I'm important too. Please make me feel wanted, unconditionally loved and needed."

"Okay, Jussie, you can run away from home," I tenderly whispered as I started picking out clothes. "Well, we'll need pj's, your coat . . ."

"Mama," he said, "what are you doin'?"

"We'll also need my coat and nightgown." I packed these items into a bag and placed them by the front door. "Okay, Jussie, are you sure you want to run away from home?"

"Yeah, but where are you goin'?"

"Well, if you're going to run away from home, then Mama's going with you, because I would never want you to be alone. I love you too much, Justin Carl."

We held each other while we talked. "Why do you want to come with me?"

I looked into his eyes. "Because I love you, Justin. My life would never be the same if you went away. So I want to make sure you'll be safe. If you do go, I will go with you."

"Can Daddy come?"

"No, Daddy has to stay home with your brothers, Erickson and Trevor, and Daddy has to work and take care of the house while we're gone."

"Can Freddi [the hamster] come?"

"No, Freddi has to stay here, too."

He thought for a while and said, "Mama, can we stay home?"

"Yes, Justin, we can stay home."

"Mama,"

"Yes, Justin?"

"I love you."

"I love you too, honey. How about you help me make some popcorn?"

"All right."

In that moment I knew the wondrous gift of motherhood I had been given, that the sacred responsibilities to help develop a child's sense of security and self-esteem are nothing to be taken lightly. I realized that in my arms I held the precious gift of childhood; a beautiful piece of clay willing and wanting to be cuddled and magnificently molded into a confident adult masterpiece. I learned that as a mother I should never "run away" from the opportunity to show my children they are wanted, important, lovable and the most precious gift from God.

Lois Krueger

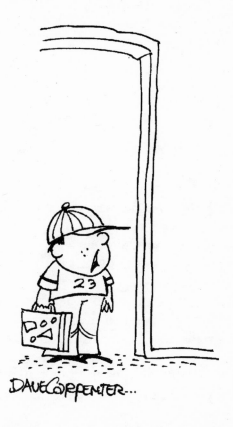

"I said I'm running away! Shouldn't somebody be warming up the car?"

Reprinted with permission from Dave Carpenter.

Taking a Break

Being a working woman can be tough, but holding a job and having children is even tougher.

There's a story about a mother with three active boys who were playing cops and robbers in the back yard after dinner one summer evening.

One of the boys "shot" his mother and yelled, "Bang, you're dead." She slumped to the ground and when she didn't get up right away, a neighbor ran over to see if she had been hurt in the fall.

When the neighbor bent over, the overworked mother opened one eye and said, "Shhh. Don't give me away. It's the only chance I get to rest."

The Best of Bits & Pieces

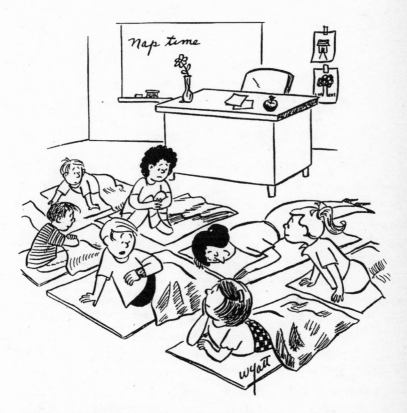

"Well, somebody better wake her up. It's past time to go home."

Reprinted with permission from Peggy Andy Wyatt.

Help Wanted—The Ideal Mother

The transition into motherhood can be tough on anyone.

"I just wasn't cut out to be a good mother," says the weary voice of my friend on the telephone. "I can't get the baby to sleep through the night. I scream too much at my toddler when he gets into things. And my six-year-old is always whining that she doesn't have enough to do. At least in the office I have someone to teach me the job and my evenings and weekends off."

I understand her completely because I am also a mother. The difficulty isn't just that first transition, either. It's the ongoing reshaping of pieces of a personality and a way of living to become the kind of mother a child needs at each stage of his or her life.

For example, a job description for the kind of person who would be an ideal mother for a baby might read like this:

Wanted—Easygoing, relaxed, loving type to care for infant. Should enjoy rocking, cuddling, be able to hold baby patiently for 20-minute feedings every three or four hours without fidgeting. Light sleeper, early riser. No degree necessary. Must take all shifts, seven-day week. No vacation unless can arrange to have own mother as temporary substitute. No opportunity to advance.

A year and a half later, the ideal candidate for the job of mothering the same child would match this description:

Wanted—Athlete in top condition to safeguard tireless toddler. Needs quick reflexes, boundless energy, infinite patience. ESP helpful. Knowledge of first aid essential. Must be able to drive, cook, phone, work despite constant distractions. Workday, 15 hours. No coffee or lunch breaks unless child naps. Would consider pediatric nurse with Olympic background.

In another 18 months, the same mother should be able to meet these qualifications:

Position Open—Expert in early childhood education to provide stimulating, loving, creative, individualized learning environment for pre-schooler. Should have experience in art, music, recreation, be able to speak one foreign language. Training in linguistics, psychology and Montessori desirable. Two hours off five days a week when nursery school is in session and child is well.

Job stability improves somewhat when a child is between 6 and 12, and the mothers who cope most easily meet these qualifications:

Good Opportunity—For expert in recreation, camping, Indian arts, all sports. Should be able to referee. Must be willing to be den mother, room mother, block mother. Public relations skills essential. Should be able to deal effectively with teachers, PTA officers, other parents. Knowledge of sex education, new math required. Must have no objections to mud, insect collections, pets, neighbor's kids.

A mother changes occupations again when her child reaches 13 or 14 and must face up to new requirements:

Job Available—For specialist in adolescent psychology, with experience in large-quantity cooking. Tolerance is chief requirement. Slight hearing loss helpful or must provide own ear plugs. Must be unflappable. Should be able to sense when presence is embarrassing to child and disappear.

After 18 years as a working mother, a woman is qualified for only one more job:

Urgently Needed—Financier to provide money, clothes, music, wheels to collegian. No advice necessary. Position may last indefinitely. Ample time left to take income-producing work.

Like most want ads, there are some things these work descriptions leave out: (1) A mother who has more than one child must usually hold down two or more of these posts simultaneously; (2) those who handle the jobs best work themselves permanently out of a job, and (3) there are greater rewards than anyone could ever imagine.

Joan Beck
Submitted by Jeanette Lisefski

THE FAMILY CIRCUS

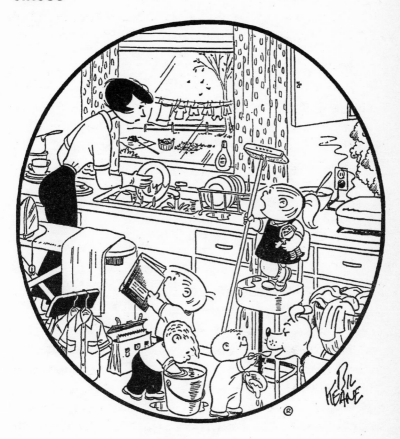

"You used to WORK before you were married, didn't you, Mommy?"

Reprinted with special permission of King Features Syndicate.

Graduation Day

A mother *is not a person to lean on but a person to make leaning unnecessary.*

Dorothy Canfield Fisher

Today Cathy will be going to kindergarten. Cathy is my youngest and I am feeling nostalgic. If I had the courage to admit it, I'd say I'm feeling sad and a little scared. Why am I feeling this way? I didn't feel sad when Renata, her older sister, went to school. Why, I was excited and rejoiced about her new freedom.

It seems like yesterday that Cathy was such a quiet, contented baby. She was always a real joy to have around. She played quietly with her stuffed animals or our family dog. She and the dog loved to hide together under the blanket tent I'd throw over the big lounge chair.

Her life and mine would dramatically change now. She would be part of the world out there. I would have a harder time protecting her from the bumps and scrapes of life.

Perhaps I was being overprotective now because Cathy had been diagnosed at three as having a rare disease. No one but the family knew or even saw anything different about her.

I'm about to leave the kitchen to awaken Cathy for her big day. But here she comes, all bright eyes and smiles, dressed in a new red plaid skirt and blouse. She gives me a big hug as we say our good mornings.

"Good morning, you're up early!" I greet her.

"Morning, Mom," is mumbled into my apron because of her big hug. "See Mom, I got dressed all by myself and even brushed my hair." She proudly twirls a pirouette to show me.

"But I can't put this ribbon in my hair." She hands me the brush, rubber band and red ribbon. I am amazed at how efficient she is this particular morning.

As I tend to her hair and ribbon, I ask her once more, "Would you like me to walk you to school this first day?"

I get the same answer as yesterday, "No, Mom, I can find my way all by myself. Renata, Leslie and I walked to the school yesterday and they showed me how to find the path through the woods right to the playground.

"And Mom, they have it all finished now and everything is brand new—the slide, swings and basketball hoops. It's going to be great!"

My reply to her enthusiasm is, "Stand still so I can finish your hair ribbon."

Then I gently push her toward the table. She quickly slides into her chair and attacks her breakfast. I turn back to the kitchen cupboards and take a deep breath, but it doesn't melt the lump in my throat or dull the ache in my chest.

I glance at the clock. "You can't leave before 8:30, so just slow down and chew your food."

In a few minutes she has finished the last drop of milk. Without prompting, she goes off to brush her teeth and comes back with her sweater.

"Is it time to go now?" she pleads.

"When this hand reaches 6," I point out to her on the clock.

I tentatively venture for the umpteenth time, "You're sure you don't want me to walk you to school?"

"No, Mom, I want to go alone." She goes out onto the deck to call to the dog and check the back yard.

"Is it time now?" She is hopping up and down.

With a sigh, I say, "Yes, dear."

I give her a big lingering hug, and off she races down the split-level stairs and out the front door. Standing at the top of our stairs, I can watch through the window. She is running down the sidewalk. Then suddenly she stops, turns and races back toward the house. "Oh, no," I think, expecting to have to change out of slippers for a walk to school after all.

The front door bangs open and up the stairs she flies to throw her little arms around me and press her cheek into my tummy. The long tight hug ends as she turns her eyes up to mine and seriously proclaims, "You'll be all right, Mom. I'll be home at noon."

Then off she dashes into her new world of school adventures, excited and happy to be graduating from babyhood. My misty eyes follow her progress to the end of our walk. She turns around again and waves to me. I wave back and find I can now smile.

The lump in my chest has melted as I think about her display of love. Yes, I will be all right as I go on to my own adventures. This is my graduation day, too.

Mary Ann Detzler

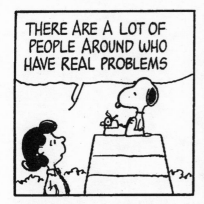

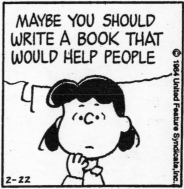

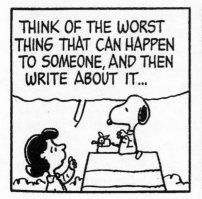

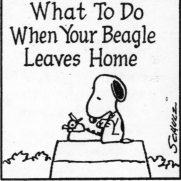

PEANUTS. Reprinted by permission of United Feature Syndicate, Inc.

A Mother's Letter to the World

Dear World:

My son starts school today. It's going to be strange and new to him for a while. And I wish you would sort of treat him gently.

You see, up to now, he's been king of the roost. He's been boss of the back yard. I have always been around to repair his wounds, and to soothe his feelings.

But now—things are going to be different.

This morning, he's going to walk down the front steps, wave his hand and start on his great adventure that will probably include wars and tragedy and sorrow.

To live his life in the world he has to live in will require faith and love and courage.

So, World, I wish you would sort of take him by his young hand and teach him the things he will have to know. Teach him—but gently, if you can. Teach him that for every scoundrel there is a hero; that for every crooked politician there is a dedicated leader; that for every enemy there is a friend. Teach him the wonders of books.

Give him quiet time to ponder the eternal mystery of birds in the sky, bees in the sun, and flowers on the green hill. Teach him it is far more honorable to fail than to cheat.

Teach him to have faith in his own ideas, even if everyone else tells him they are wrong. Teach him to sell his brawn and brains to the highest bidder, but never to put a price on his heart and soul.

Teach him to close his ears to a howling mob . . . and to stand and fight if he thinks he's right.

Teach him gently, World, but don't coddle him, because only the test of fire makes fine steel.

This is a big order, World, but see what you can do. He's such a nice little fellow.

Author Unknown

To Give the Gift of Life

You had your eyes open a little while ago, but now you just want to sleep. I wish you would open your eyes and look at me. My child, my precious, my angel sent from heaven . . . this will be the last time we are together. As I hold you close to me and feel your tiny body warm against my own, I look at you and look at you . . . I feel as if my eyes can't hold enough of you. For a human being so small, there is a lot of you to look at . . . in such a short time. In a few minutes, they will come and take you away from me. But for now, this is our time together and you belong to only me.

Your cheeks are still bruised from your birth—they feel so soft to my fingertip, like the wing of a butterfly. Your eyebrows are tightly clenched in concentration—are you dreaming? You have too many eyelashes to count and yet I want to engrave them all in my mind. I don't want to forget anything about you. Is it all right that you are breathing so rapidly? I don't know anything about babies—maybe I never will. But I know one thing for sure—I love you with all my heart. I love you so much and there is no way to tell you. I hope that someday you will understand. I am giving you away because I love you. I want you to have in your life all the things I could never have in mine—safety, compassion, joy and acceptance. I want you to be loved for who you are.

I wish I could squish you back inside of me—I'm not ready to let you go. If I could just hold you like this forever and never have to face tomorrow—would everything be all right? No, I know everything will only be all right if I let you go. I just didn't expect to feel this way—I didn't know you would be so beautiful and so perfect. I feel as if my heart is being pulled from my body right through my skin. I didn't know I would feel so much pain.

Tomorrow your mom and dad are coming to the hospital to pick you up, and you will start your life. I pray that they will tell you about me. I hope they will know how brave I have been. I hope they will tell you how much I loved you because I won't be around to tell you myself. I will cry every day somewhere inside of me because I will miss you so much. I hope I will see you again someday— but I want you to grow up to be strong and beautiful and to have everything you want. I want you to have a home and a family. I want you to have children of your own someday that are as beautiful as you are. I hope that you will try to understand and not be angry with me.

The nurse comes into the room and reaches out her arms for you. Do I have to let you go? I can feel your heart beating rapidly and you finally open your eyes. You look into my eyes with trust and innocence, and we lock hearts. I give you to the nurse. I feel as if I could die. Good-bye, my baby—a piece of my heart will be with you always and forever. I love you, I love you . . . I love you . . .

Patty Hansen

Mother's Day

One day while in my early 30s, I sat in a Midwestern church and burst into tears. It was Mother's Day, and ladies of all shapes and sizes, young and old, were being applauded by their families and the whole congregation. Each received a lovely rose and returned to the pews, where I sat empty-handed. Sorry to my soul, I was convinced I had missed my chance at that great adventure, that selective sorority called "motherhood."

All that changed one February when, pushing 40 and pushing with all my might, I brought forth Gabriel Zacharias. It took 24 hours of labor for me to produce that little four-pound, eight-ounce bundle of joy. No wonder those ladies got flowers!

Any mother who has survived one birth amazes herself at her willingness to go for two. Jordan Raphael was born the following March. He was smaller and labor was shorter; but I still felt I deserved flowers.

The sorority I joined requires an extended hazing period: nine months of demanding cravings for unusual foods you can't keep down; weight gain you can't explain; a walk that is part buffalo and part duck; unique bedtime constructions of pillows designed to support this bulge and fill in that gap but avoid all pressure on the bladder; and extensive stretch marks culminating in excruciating labor pain.

With labor, the hazing period ends. But with the child's birth, the initiation period in this great sorority has just begun. The painful tugs on the heart strings far exceed whatever physical pain labor required. There was my older son's first cut that drew blood, his spiked fevers, his long bout with pneumonia; my younger son's terror at a big barking dog, his near-miss with a car, the death of his pet rat.

While the hazing period may seem overlong, this initiation period never ends. I wake up when my sons cough. I hear their teddy bears land with a soft thud on the floor next to their beds. In the supermarket I respond to children calling "Mo-ther!" and the kids, I realize, aren't even my own!

I've advanced past bottle weaning, potty training, the first days of school and the first trip to the dentist. Coming up are first crushes, first heartbreaks, and first times behind the wheel of a car. I hope to someday see them each happily married with children of their own. Then I will gain entry into that even more exclusive sorority of "grandmotherhood."

For now, the password to my heart is "Mom," and I thank my sons for this. Especially on the days of their birth, happily on a special Sunday in May. My young sons do not yet realize how much I value this remarkable membership and won't note it with flowers unless prompted. Yet every time we take a walk, they pluck me a short-stemmed blossom, "just because."

This year I look forward to celebrating Mother's Day— the divine achievement of the physical, the grand acceptance of the commonplace, the exquisite gratitude of watching my sons become uniquely themselves. Because of Gabriel and Jordan, I am a dues-paying, card-carrying member of The Club. Happy Mother's Day to me!

Sharon Nicola Cramer

THE FAMILY CIRCUS

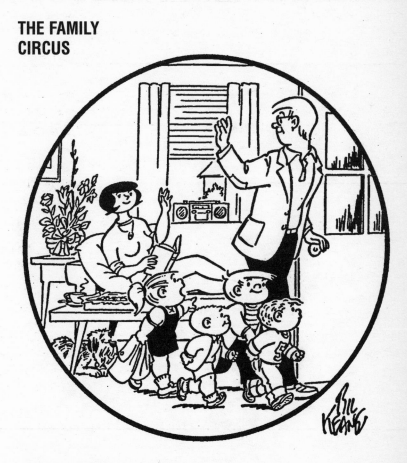

"Poor Mommy. We get to go to the movies for Mother's Day and she has to stay home."

Reprinted with special permission of King Feature Syndicate, Inc.

6

SPECIAL
MOMENTS

Today a new sun rises for me; everything lives, everything is animated, everything seems to speak to me of my passion, everything invites me to cherish it . . .

Anne de Lenclos

In a Hurry

The work will wait while you show the child the rainbow, but the rainbow won't wait while you do the work.

Patricia Clafford

I was in a hurry.

I came rushing through our dining room in my best suit, focused on getting ready for an evening meeting. Gillian, my four-year-old, was dancing about to one of her favorite oldies, "Cool," from *West Side Story*.

I was in a hurry, on the verge of being late. Yet a small voice inside of me said, *Stop*.

So I stopped. I looked at her. I reached out, grabbed her hand and spun her around. My seven-year-old, Caitlin, came into our orbit, and I grabbed her, too. The three of us did a wild jitterbug around the dining room and into the living room. We were laughing. We were spinning. Could the neighbors see the lunacy through the windows? It didn't matter. The song ended with a dramatic flourish and our dance finished with it. I patted them on their bottoms and sent them to take their baths.

They went up the stairs, gasping for breath, their giggles bouncing off the walls. I went back to business. I was bent over, shoving papers into my briefcase, when I overheard my youngest say to her sister, "Caitlin, isn't Mommy the bestest one?"

I froze. How close I had come to hurrying through life, missing that moment. My mind went to the awards and diplomas that covered the walls of my office. No award, no achievement I have ever earned can match this: *Isn't Mommy the bestest one?*

My child said that at age four. I don't expect her to say it at age 14. But at age 40, if she bends down over that pine box to say good-bye to the cast-off container of my soul, I want her to say it then.

Isn't Mommy the bestest one?

It doesn't fit on my résumé. But I want it on my tombstone.

Gina Barrett Schlesinger

No Small Act of Kindness

If I can stop one Heart from breaking,
I shall not live in vain;
If I can ease one Life the Aching,
Or cool one pain,
Or help one fainting Robin
Unto his Nest again,
I shall not live in vain.

Emily Dickinson

The day was Thankful Thursday, our "designated day" of service. It's a weekly tradition that my two little girls and I began years ago. Thursday has become our day to go out in the world and make a positive contribution. On this particular Thursday, we had no idea exactly what we were going to do, but we knew that something would present itself.

Driving along a busy Houston road, praying for guidance in our quest to fulfill our weekly Act of Kindness, the noon hour appropriately triggered hunger pangs in my two little ones. They wasted no time in letting me know, chanting, "McDonald's, McDonald's, McDonald's" as we drove along. I relented and began searching earnestly for the nearest McDonald's. Suddenly I realized that almost every intersection I passed through was occupied by a panhandler. And then it hit me! If my two little ones were hungry, then all these panhandlers must be hungry, too. Perfect! Our Act of Kindness had presented itself. We were going to buy lunch for the panhandlers.

After finding a McDonald's and ordering two Happy Meals for my girls, I ordered an additional 15 lunches and we set out to deliver them. It was exhilarating. We would pull alongside a panhandler, make a contribution, and tell him or her that we hoped things got better. Then we'd say, "Oh, by the way . . . here's lunch." And then we would varoom off to the next intersection.

It was the best way to give. There wasn't enough time for us to introduce ourselves or explain what we were going to do, nor was there time for them to say anything back to us. The Act of Kindness was anonymous and empowering for each of us, and we loved what we saw in the rear view mirror: a surprised and delighted person holding up his lunch bag and just looking at us as we drove off. It was wonderful!

We had come to the end of our "route" and there was a small woman standing there, asking for change. We handed her our final contribution and lunch bag, and then immediately made a U-turn to head back in the opposite direction for home. Unfortunately, the light caught us again and we were stopped at the same inter-section where this little woman stood. I was embarrassed and didn't know quite how to behave. I didn't want her to feel obligated to say or do anything.

She made her way to our car, so I put the window down just as she started to speak. "No one has ever done any-thing like this for me before," she said with amazement. I replied, "Well, I'm glad that we were the first." Feeling uneasy, and wanting to move the conversation along, I asked, "So, when do you think you'll eat your lunch?"

She just looked at me with her huge, tired brown eyes and said, "Oh honey, I'm not going to eat *this* lunch." I was confused, but before I could say anything, she continued. "You see, I have a little girl of my own at home and she just *loves* McDonald's, but I can never buy it for her because I just don't have the money. But you know what . . . tonight *she* is going to have McDonald's!"

I don't know if the kids noticed the tears in my eyes. So many times I had questioned whether our Acts of Kindness were too small or insignificant to really effect change. Yet in that moment, I recognized the truth of Mother Teresa's words: "We cannot do great things—only small things with great love."

Donna Wick

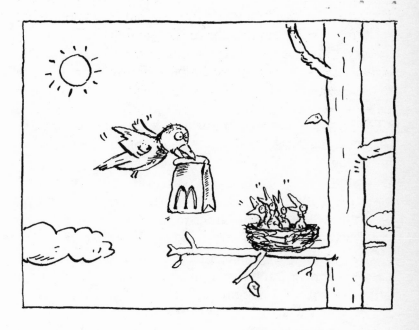

Copyright ©1987 by David Sipress. Reprinted by permission of HarperCollins Publishers, Inc.

The Last Jar of Jelly

Our children grew up on peanut butter and jelly sand-wiches. Even my husband and I sometimes sneak one in late at night with a glass of milk. I believe that the Earl of Sandwich himself would agree with me that the success of this universally loved concoction lies not in the brand of peanut butter used, but rather in the jelly. The right jelly delights the palate, and homemade is the only choice.

I wasn't the jelly maker in this family. My mother-in-law was. She didn't provide a wide range of flavors, either. It was either grape or blackberry. This limited choice was a welcome relief in the days of toddlers, sib-lings and puppies. When all around me other decisions and choices had to be made, making peanut butter and jelly sandwiches was easy. And since we liked both fla-vors, we usually picked whatever jar was at the front of the pantry or refrigerator.

The only contribution I made to the jelly making was to save baby food jars, which my mother-in-law would fill with the tasty gel, seal with wax and send back home with us. For the past 22 years of my married life, when-ever I wanted to make a peanut butter and jelly sandwich for myself or my husband or one of the children, all I had to do was reach for one of those little jars of jelly. It was always there. Jelly making was just a way of life for my mother-in-law. She always did it, following the same rituals—from picking the fruit to setting the finished jelly on the homemade shelves in her little pantry off the kitchen.

My father-in-law died several years ago and this past December, my mother-in-law also passed away. Among the things in the house to be divided by her children were the remaining canned goods in the pantry. Each of her children chose from the many jars of tomato juice, green beans and jelly. When my husband brought his jars home, we carefully put them away in our pantry.

The other day I reached in there to retrieve jelly for a quick sandwich, and there it was. Sitting all alone on the far side of the shelf was a small jar of grape jelly. The lid was somewhat rusty in places. Written on it with a black marker was "GR" for grape and the year the jelly had been made.

As I picked up the jar, I suddenly realized something that I had failed to see earlier. I reopened the pantry door to be sure. Yes, this was it, this was the last jar of "Memommie jelly." We would always have store-bought jelly, but this was the last jar we would ever have from the patient, loving hands of my mother-in-law. Although she had been gone for nearly a year, so much of her had remained with us. We hardly ever opened a jar of jelly at the breakfast table without kidding about those thousands of little jars she had filled. Our children had never known a day without their grandmother's jelly. It seems like such a small thing, and most days it was something that was taken for granted. But today it seemed a great treasure.

Holding that last jar in my hand, my heart traveled back to meeting my mother-in-law for the first time. I could see her crying on our wedding day, and later, kissing and loving our children as if she didn't have five other grandchildren. I could see her walking the fields of the farm, patiently waiting while others tended to the cows. I could see her walking in the woods or riding the hay wagon behind the tractor. I saw her face as it looked when we surprised her by meeting her at church. I saw her caring for a sick spouse and surrounded by loving children at the funeral.

I put the jelly back on the shelf. No longer was it just a jar of jelly. It was the end of a family tradition. I guess I believed that as long as it was there, a part of my mother-in-law would always live on.

We have many things that once belonged to my husband's parents. There are guns, tools, handmade sweaters and throws, and some furniture. We have hundreds of pictures and many more memories. These are the kinds of things that you expect to survive the years and to pass on to your children. But I'm just not ready to give up this last jelly jar, and all the memories its mere presence allows me to hold onto. The jar of jelly won't keep that long. It will either have to be eaten or thrown out . . . but not today.

Andy Skidmore

A Christmas Story

It was just a few more days until Christmas in San Francisco, and the shopping downtown was starting to get to us. I remember crowds of people waiting impatiently for slow-moving buses and streetcars on those little cement islands in the middle of the street. Most of us were loaded down with packages, and it looked like many of us were beginning to wonder if all those countless friends and relatives actually *deserved* so many gifts in the first place. This was not the Christmas spirit I'd been raised with.

When I finally found myself virtually shoved up the steps of a jammed streetcar, the idea of standing there packed like a sardine the whole way home was almost more than I could take. What I would have given for a seat! I must have been in some kind of exhausted daze because as people gradually got off, it took me a while to notice that there was room to breathe again.

Then I saw something out of the corner of my eye. A small, dark-skinned boy—he couldn't have been more than five or six—tugged on a woman's sleeve and asked, "Would you like a seat?" He quietly led her to the closest free seat he could find. Then he set out to find another tired person. As soon as each rare, new seat became available, he would quickly move through the crowd in search of another burdened woman who desperately needed to rest her feet.

When I finally felt the tug on my own sleeve, I was absolutely dazzled by the beauty in this little boy's eyes. He took my hand, saying, "Come with me," and I think I'll remember that smile as long as I live. As I happily placed my heavy load of packages on the floor, the little emissary of love immediately turned to help his next subject.

The people on the streetcar, as usual, had been studiously avoiding each other's eyes, but now they began to exchange shy glances and smiles. A businessman offered a section of newspaper to the stranger next to him; three people stooped to return a gift that had tumbled to the floor. And now people were speaking to one another. That little boy had tangibly changed something—we all relaxed into a subtle feeling of warmth and actually enjoyed the trip through the final stops along the route.

I didn't notice when the child got off. I looked up at one point and he was gone. When I reached my stop I practically floated off that streetcar, wishing the driver a happy holiday, noticing the sparkling Christmas lights on my street in a fresh, new way. Or maybe I was seeing them in an old way, with the same open wonder I felt when *I* was five or six. I thought, "So *that's* what they mean by *And a little child shall lead them. . . .*"

Beverly M. Bartlett

Who Won?

I saw a beautiful example of kindness in 1968 during the Special Olympics track and field meet. One participant was Kim Peek, a brain-damaged, severely handicapped boy racing in the 50-yard dash.

Kim was racing against two other athletes with cerebral palsy. They were in wheelchairs; Kim was the lone runner. As the gun sounded, Kim moved quickly ahead of the other two. Twenty yards ahead and 10 yards from the finish line, he turned to see how the others were coming. The girl had turned her wheelchair around and was stuck against the wall. The other boy was pushing his wheelchair backward with his feet. Kim stopped, went back and pushed the little girl across the finish line. The boy in the wheelchair going backward won the race. The girl took second. Kim lost.

Or did he? The crowd that gave Kim a standing ovation didn't think so.

Dan Clark

Bush Sneakers

I was already nervous. There I was, standing in line at a White House state dinner—yes, that White House—about to shake hands with President and Mrs. Bush, trying to hold my smile in place and think of something intelligent to say. Lost in my thoughts, I heard my husband's voice. "Oh, Christine would love to make her a pair." I looked up just in time to see the president staring down at my husband's shoes. The dark, hand-painted tennis shoes were not what most people would expect to find as the accompanying foot gear for a tuxedo. Over the years, while my husband, Wally Amos, was out promoting his "famous" chocolate chip cookies, I'd created unique works of art on his clothes, including my most recent venture into footwear.

The next few seconds remain a blur to this day, but the upshot is that Wally volunteered me to paint a pair of sneakers for the president's wife, Barbara. My first reaction was, "Thanks, honey. Maybe you'd like to handle all the household chores for a week while I create executive sneakers," followed by the assumption that it was all small talk, and wasn't it nice that the president of the

United States had noticed my husband's sneakers. Nevertheless, a week later a special delivery package from the White House arrived with a pair of the first lady's sneakers for me to paint on and a "knock yourself out" note. *Oh well,* I thought to myself, *it is for the first lady.*

Of course, once I realized that this was real, I completely got into it. I painted pictures of Millie the dog, the grandkids, books (for Mrs. Bush's support of literacy), rainbows, suns, palm trees—on the tongues, the sides, the laces. Those shoes were truly works of art by the time they winged their way back to Washington, and I was proud of them.

Suddenly, I found myself checking the mail on a regular basis to see what the response was. A few weeks later, I got a very warm, handwritten note from the first lady, thanking me profusely and telling me how wonderful the shoes were.

But it didn't end there. Months later, my husband was back at the White House for a library luncheon at which Mrs. Bush was to speak. Just before the luncheon, when she found out that Wally was to be in attendance, Mrs. Bush had an aide get the magic tennies. She put them on, had pictures taken with Wally—of course he had his on—and then kept them on for the luncheon. There stood Mrs. Bush, with her dignified first lady attire, and her newly painted tennis shoes. I was thrilled again.

My outgoing husband is always seizing an opportunity. This time, he gets my thanks for making a lasting memory for me. I hope those bright and cheery sneakers are still in the Bush closet somewhere—that is, if Millie hasn't used them for chew toys by now.

Christine Harris-Amos with Cliff Marsh

Feather Light

And all the loveliest things there be come simply, so it seems to me.

Edna St. Vincent Millay

In fifth grade I sat at a desk third row from the left, second seat in front, with my hands folded and my feet on the floor. Pastor Beikman served up the commandments every morning and we learned to chew them, swallow them and fear them. This was the essence of my early education: study, memorize, recite. Parochial school grounded me in uniforms and conventions, in a world of curriculum where men were cherished and women were invisible. Men discovered new lands, explained the laws of the universe and wrote the Bible. But it was a woman who quickened my soul and invited me to look deeply at life, to love sincerely and to see God in everything.

One morning the pastor announced he was changing duties and leaving the school staff. He introduced us to our replacement teacher, Miss Newhart, and a ripple of excitement filled the room. A tall woman with a beehive hairdo, platform shoes and a skirt that almost showed her knees, Miss Newhart was powerful and light all at once. Her hands, big and freckled like a robin's breast, spoke with gestures large enough to fill the air around us. From a sack the size of a suitcase, she handed a feather to each student and told us they were gifts from their original owners—birds who'd cast off their excess plumage and left behind the things they no longer needed to carry. That morning our world changed, and soon, so too would we.

In history class that day, Miss Newhart told the story of Christopher Columbus. Having been at sea too long, the sailors on his ship became restive and demanded a port. There was talk of mutiny, and Columbus was said to have feared for his life. Then one morning, a feather floated down from the sky above, a sign that land was near. Miss Newhart said the sailors spied more gulls, screeching and whirling in the air, then quite dramatically she flung out her arms and the plump, freckled skin of her triceps quivered just a bit. She turned quick circles so that her skirt flung out flapping at her thighs and her feet went round fast. I thought she, too, might lift up and fly. She helped me see what those sailors must have seen: there is hope even in the smallest of things.

The next morning, Miss Newhart's sack was bulging at the seams. Inside it there was a poster of *The Last Supper*, a paintbrush, a compass and a long cylindrical tube. From the tube she pulled out a black and white drawing and tacked it on the particle board. It was a circle with a man inside, his arms stretched wide against the circumference, feet splayed at the bottom; dimensions, figures, designs and numbers were scrawled across the sheet. "Da Vinci," she said in a whisper, "was more than a painter. He studied subjects until he knew them well: man, nature, science, math . . ."

"Did he know anything about feathers?" I asked. The woman with the beehive hairdo loved that question.

A pioneer in the science of aerodynamics, Leonardo da Vinci studied feathers. When viewed from the top, a feather appears convex, arched delicately up and out, allowing the air to flow over it without resistance. When feathers are put together, as a wing, they create an airfoil, something that provides just the right resistance against the air as it moves through the feathers. Miss Newhart, who was more than a teacher, and da Vinci, who was more than a painter, showed me how to see the extraordinary in a small thing.

Later that day, Miss Newhart took us beyond the confines of the school walls to a nearby field, wide and high with weeds. There we lay among the blonde grasses and covered our bodies with sticks, leaves and stalks. These became our nests, windows to the sky. Hidden there we learned to be quiet, to rest and watch, to let the bugs crawl over and beyond us, to listen for the birds and study their movements.

In the afternoon, Miss Newhart stood at the door as we were leaving, touched each of us on the shoulder and said "Good-bye" or "God bless." I remember how warm and light her hands were. She often asked me to stay awhile, to straighten the chairs, put away ruffled papers, and dust chalk from the board. During one of those grace-filled afternoons, I shared a troubled thought I had been keeping secret. I told Miss Newhart that I might love birds more than I loved God, a sin according to the commandments. My teacher rummaged through her cluttered desk, found her Bible, flipped it open to the Psalms and read, "He will cover you with His feathers, and under His wings you will find refuge; His faithfulness will be your shield and rampart." She wrote down the little verse and handed it to me. I have it still. I didn't know what rampart meant—it didn't really matter—but something deep inside of me awakened: I was given full permission to love things deeply, for God was in all things and had given them to me. On the way home that afternoon I imagined I could fly. I ran full speed, arms outstretched and legs behind me, skimming the sidewalks as though I were a bird.

Around my neck I wear a gold charm—a bird, given to me when I was younger. That bird's wings have become my symbol. They remind me of those sidewalks I flew over all those years before, and of the roads I've traveled since. And I have become more of a feather myself as the years have flown by: I am less resistant to what life offers up, and the pressures flow over me much more easily. As a teacher, I've guided children through the sometimes rough waters of fractions, spelling lessons and self-doubt. I have led them to safe shores when they were lost. I've learned to rest in quiet places now and then, and to leave behind the things I no longer need to carry, like grudges, sorrows and regrets. I have an inner strength, a gentle state of being, and I believe with all my heart no rampart will thwart me.

Melody Arnett

365 Days

According to my friends and associates, I'm secure, educated, modestly intelligent, organized and creative. But for most of my adult life, for 14 days out of each year, I felt exactly the opposite of those attributes. What brought this on, you ask? Not PMS, but worse—my parents' annual visit. Being separated from them by 1,600 miles for 351 days a year, I got on with my life quite well, being wife, mother, volunteer and businesswoman. But my parents' annual visits were excruciating for me.

The story is an old one—the first-born child who could never live up to her father's expectations. In the eyes of others I was pleasantly successful in my endeavors, but not to Dad. And I spent most of my life resenting him for that, and deep in my psyche, resenting myself.

Not only did I suffer during my parents' visits, but so did everyone around me. Certainly my sweet husband of 32 years, Dave, suffered along with me. For weeks before the visit, I'd scour the house, nag my husband to do little fix-up jobs, buy new drapes, pillows, sheets—and generally turn our household budget on its ear. I'd plan gourmet meals, bake till the freezer was full and hound my children about rooms, etiquette and raising their voices. During the visit, an ever-present aura of tension surrounded me like a gossamer veil. (Maybe it was more like a wet, wool blanket!) After the visit, nights of discussions with my hubby ensued. I would try to decipher what was, and wasn't, said by my father. And I would cry myself to sleep, inconsolable, the child of rejection and exhaustion. Thirty-two years of marriage can have its ups and downs, but the one *real* test of Dave's love was helping me survive those visits!

When I reached my 40s, immortality (or the lack of it) began to rear its nagging little head. I'd been into the study of spirituality for several years, sort of a peripheral investigation of ideas. I was a closet psychic, not about to acknowledge it publicly. However, every year for 14 days, my spirituality deserted me, and I was left as naked, defenseless and vulnerable as a five-year-old child.

Then one year Dad was diagnosed with Parkinson's disease. In a short time he turned from the vital, intelligent, athletic god of my childhood into a stumbling, gaunt, confused old man. With the clock ticking faster than ever for both of us, I came to the realization that before Dad left this life, I had to mend our broken relationship and let go of my feelings about never living up to his expectations. But how? I'd tried everything I could think of. The only thing left was to forgive him.

So I did. Just saying aloud, "I forgive you," changed my whole inner experience from self-doubt to peacefulness. I let go of "should have," "could have" and "I wish." In the process I forgave me, too.

I never told my dad that I had forgiven him, but it must have been apparent to him on some level because our entire relationship changed.

The summer before Dad died, he came alone to stay with us for two weeks in August. On my part, there was no maniacal cleaning or sheet buying or tension. Because I had forgiven him, I could now talk with him as a friend and a companion—not as a resentful, disappointed, wounded daughter. We talked about his life, marriage and war experiences, and about his love of trees and animals. For the first time in our lives, he told me he admired my intuitiveness and intelligence, and how he loved the feel of our home and the beautiful gardens we grew. Together we explored some alternative healing techniques and he shared some startling psychic events that had occurred in his life. Most stunning of all, he told me for the first time that he loved me.

My father never came to my home again. After he died, my mother had a video shot with pictures of Dad's lifetime, complete with music. I see the video case now, as I look up from my writing, tucked into the bookshelf. I've never watched it. My life with my father was two weeks in August. My memories are of Dad, sitting in the wicker chair on the porch, amidst streams of sunshine and over-flowing flowerpots, joking, talking, sharing—and loving me.

Complete and unconditional forgiveness brought me soul-soothing peace and opened the door to a life I never dreamed possible.

Now, in addition to being wife, mother, grammy and psychic counselor, I'm a *whole person* 365 days a year.

Rosemarie Giessinger

Spots of a Different Color

"Honey, someone left a coat in your mother's closet," I called to my husband. The faux-leopard jacket was tucked in the back of the closet against the wall, out of place among the dark coats and sweaters. I wondered who would hide clothes in my mother-in-law's closet. We were there to get a winter coat for her because she was coming home from the hospital, a week after being rushed to the emergency room.

"Coat? What coat?" My husband looked up from sorting the mail. I took out the jacket, holding it up in the light for him to see. "Oh, that jacket. Mom bought it years ago, when I was a kid . . . you know, when they were fashionable. She and Pop even argued about getting it."

I thought of the woman I'd known for 30 years. She bought her housedresses and polyester pantsuits at Kmart or Sears, kept her gray hair tightly confined in a hair net and chose the smallest piece of meat on the dinner platter when it was passed around the table. I knew she wasn't the kind of flamboyant type who would own a faux-leopard print jacket.

"I can't imagine Mom wearing this," I said to him.

"I don't think she ever wore it outside the house," my husband answered.

Removing the jacket from its padded hanger, I carried it to her bed and laid it on the white chenille bedspread. It seemed to sprawl like an exotic animal. My hands brushed the thick, plush fur, and the spots changed luster as my fingers sank into the pile.

My husband stood at the door. "I used to see Mom run her fingers over the fur, just like you are," he said.

As I slid my arms into the sleeves, the jacket released a perfume of gardenias and dreams. It swung loose from my shoulders, its high collar brushing my cheeks, the faux fur soft as velvet. It belonged to a glamorous, bygone era, the days of Lana Turner and Joan Crawford, but not in the closet of the practical 83-year-old woman I knew.

"Why didn't you tell me Mom had a leopard jacket?" I whispered, but my husband had left the room to water the plants.

If I'd been asked to make a list of items my mother-in-law would never want in her life, that jacket would have been near the top. Yet finding it changed our relationship. It made me realize how little I knew about this woman's hopes and dreams. We took it to the hospital for her to wear home. She blushed when she saw it, and turned even rosier at the gentle teasing of the staff.

In our last three years together, I bought her gifts of perfume, lotion and makeup instead of sensible under-wear and slippers. We had a lunch date once a week, where she wore her jacket, and she began to curl her hair so it would be fluffy and glamorous for our date. We spent time looking at her photo album, and I finally began to see the young woman there, with the Cupid's bow mouth.

Faux fur has come back into fashion. It appears in shop windows and on the street. Every time I catch a glimpse of it, I'm reminded of my mother-in-law's jacket, and that all of us have a secret self that needs to be encouraged and shared with those we love.

Grazina Smith

7

LIVE YOUR DREAM

Alice laughed. "There's no use trying," she said. "One can't believe impossible things." "I daresay you haven't had much practice," said the Queen. "When I was your age, I always did it for half an hour a day. Why, sometimes, I've believed as many as six impossible things before breakfast."

Lewis Carroll
Through the Looking Glass

The Wind Beneath Her Wings

Far away there in the sunshine are my highest aspirations. I may not reach them but I can look up and see their beauty, believe in them and try to follow them.

Louisa May Alcott

In 1959, when Jean Harper was in the third grade, her teacher gave the class an assignment to write a report on what they wanted to be when they grew up. Jean's father was a crop duster pilot in the little farming community in Northern California where she was raised, and Jean was totally captivated by airplanes and flying. She poured her heart into her report and included all of her dreams; she wanted to crop dust, make parachute jumps, seed clouds (something she'd seen on a TV episode of "Sky King") and be an airline pilot. Her paper came back with an "F" on it. The teacher told her it was a "fairy tale" and that none of the occupations she listed were women's jobs. Jean was crushed and humiliated.

She showed her father the paper, and he told her that of course she could become a pilot. "Look at Amelia Earhart," he said. "That teacher doesn't know what she's talking about."

But as the years went by, Jean was beaten down by the discouragement and negativity she encountered whenever she talked about her career—"Girls can't become airline pilots; never have, never will. You're not smart enough, you're crazy. That's impossible."—until finally Jean gave up.

In her senior year of high school, her English teacher was a Mrs. Dorothy Slaton. Mrs. Slaton was an uncompromising, demanding teacher with high standards and a low tolerance for excuses. She refused to treat her students like children, instead expecting them to behave like the responsible adults they would have to be to succeed in the real world after graduation. Jean was scared of her at first but grew to respect her firmness and fairness.

One day Mrs. Slaton gave the class an assignment. "What do you think you'll be doing 10 years from now?" Jean thought about the assignment. Pilot? No way. Flight attendant? I'm not pretty enough—they'd never accept me. Wife? What guy would want me? Waitress? I could do *that.* That felt safe, so she wrote it down.

Mrs. Slaton collected the papers and nothing more was said. Two weeks later, the teacher handed back the assignments, face down on each desk, and asked this question: "If you had unlimited finances, unlimited access to the finest schools, unlimited talents and abilities, what would you do?" Jean felt a rush of the old enthusiasm, and with excitement she wrote down all her old dreams. When the students stopped writing, the teacher asked, "How many students wrote the same thing on both sides of the paper?" Not one hand went up.

The next thing that Mrs. Slaton said changed the course of Jean's life. The teacher leaned forward over her desk and said, "I have a little secret for you all. You *do* have unlimited abilities and talents. You *do* have access to the finest schools, and you *can* arrange unlimited finances if you want something badly enough. This is it! When you leave school, if you don't go for your dreams, *no one* will do it for you. You can have what you want if you want it enough."

The hurt and fear of years of discouragement crumbled in the face of the truth of what Mrs. Slaton had said. Jean felt exhilarated and a little scared. She stayed after class and went up to the teacher's desk. Jean thanked Mrs. Slaton and told her about her dream of becoming a pilot. Mrs. Slaton half rose and slapped the desk top. "Then do it!" she said.

So Jean did. It didn't happen overnight. It took 10 years of hard work, facing opposition that ranged from quiet skepticism to outright hostility. It wasn't in Jean's nature to stand up for herself when someone refused or humiliated her; instead, she would quietly try to find another way.

She became a private pilot and then got the necessary ratings to fly air freight and even commuter planes, but always as a copilot. Her employers were openly hesitant about promoting her—because she was a woman. Even her father advised her to try something else. "It's impossible," he said. "Stop banging your head against the wall!"

But Jean answered, "Dad, I disagree. I believe that things are going to change, and I want to be at the head of the pack when they do."

Jean went on to do everything her third-grade teacher said was a fairy tale—she did some crop dusting, made a few hundred parachute jumps and even seeded clouds for a summer season as a weather modification pilot. In 1978, she became one of the first three female pilot trainees ever accepted by United Airlines and one of only

50 women airline pilots in the nation at the time. Today, Jean Harper is a Boeing 737 captain for United.

It was the power of one well-placed positive word, one spark of encouragement from a woman Jean respected, that gave that uncertain young girl the strength and faith to pursue her dream. Today Jean says, "I chose to believe her."

Carol Kline with Jean Harper

What Do You Want to *Be?*

*I*magination is the highest kite one can fly.

Lauren Bacall

I had one of those serendipitous moments a few weeks ago. I was in the bedroom changing one of the babies when our five-year-old, Alyssa, came and plopped down beside me on the bed.

"Mommy, what do you want to be when you grow up?" she asked.

I assumed she was playing some little imaginary game, and so to play along I responded with, "H'mmmmm. I think I would like to be a mommy when I grow up."

"You can't be that 'cause you *already* are one. What do you want to *be?*"

"Okay, maybe I will be a pastor when I grow up," I answered a second time.

"Mommy, *no,* you're *already* one of those!"

"I'm sorry, honey," I said, "but I don't understand what I'm supposed to say then."

"Mommy, just answer what you want to *be* when you grow up. You can *be anything* you want to be!"

At that point I was so moved by the experience that I could not immediately respond, and Alyssa gave up on me and left the room.

That experience—that tiny five-minute experience—touched a place deep within me. I was touched because in my daughter's young eyes, I could still be *anything* I wanted to be! My age, my present career, my five children, my husband, my bachelor's degree, my master's degree: *none of that mattered.* In her young eyes I could still dream dreams and reach for stars. In her young eyes my future was not over. In her young eyes I could still be an astronaut or a piano player or even an opera singer, perhaps. In her young eyes I still had some growing to do and a lot of "being" left in my life.

The real beauty in that encounter with my daughter was when I realized that in all her honesty and innocence, she would have asked the very same question of her grandparents and of her great-grandparent.

It has been written, "The old woman I shall become will be quite different from the woman I am now. Another I is beginning . . ."

So . . . what do you want to *be* when you grow up?

Rev. Teri Johnson

Hello, Dolly!

You gotta have a dream. If you don't have a dream, how ya gonna make a dream come true?

Bloody Mary, in the movie *South Pacific*

Music, I suppose, will be the thing that sustains me in the time of my life when I am too old for sex and not quite ready to meet God. It has always been an essential part of me. Since I have been able to form words, I have been able to rhyme them. I could catch on to anything that had a rhythm and make a song to go with it. I would take the two notes of a bobwhite in the darkness and make that the start of a song. I would latch on to the rhythm my mother made snapping beans, and before I knew it, I'd be tapping on a pot with a spoon and singing. I don't know what some of this sounded like to my family, but in my head it was beautiful music. I loved to hear the wild geese flying overhead. I would get into the music of their honking, and start to snap my fingers to their cadence and sing with them. I think I was especially drawn to them because I knew they were going somewhere. They had good reason to sing. They were free to go with the wind, to make the world their own. My song connected me to them. They took part of my spirit with them wherever they went.

When I was forced to pursue my musical dreams on my own, I would whang away at my old mandolin with the piano strings. I started getting pretty good with it, within its limitations, and people started to notice. Of course, that was exactly what I wanted. I was never one to shy away from attention. Finally, my Uncle Louis began to see that I was really serious about wanting to learn, so he taught me guitar. He gave me an old Martin guitar, and I learned the basic chords pretty quick. This was like manna from heaven to me. At last I could play along with the songs I heard in my head. Mama's family were all very musical, and I used to worry the heck out of all of them to "teach me that lick" or "play this with me." If Daddy had found it hard to get me to work in the fields before, now even he began to realize it was a fruitless undertaking.

I would sit up on top of the woodpile, playing and singing at the top of my lungs. Sometimes I would take a tobacco stake and stick it in the cracks between the boards on the front porch. A tin can on top of the tobacco stake turned it into a microphone, and the porch became my stage. I used to perform for anybody or anything I could get to watch. The younger kids left in my care would become the unwilling audience for my latest show. A two-year-old's attention span is not very long. So there I would be in the middle of my act, thinking I was really something, and my audience would start crawling away. I was so desperate to perform that on more than one occasion I sang for the chickens and the pigs and ducks. They didn't applaud much, but with the aid of a little corn, they could be counted on to hang around for a while.

Over the years, my dream for a better audience grew. I wanted to sing at the Grand Ole Opry! But people thought my chances were pretty slim and wanted to spare me a heartache, so they'd come up with answers like "You're just a kid," or "You have to be in the union" or just about anything they could think of. But I just wouldn't be denied.

You had to have a slot on the program to sing on the Opry, and there was no way I was going to get one. But finally, Jimmy C. Newman, who had a spot one Saturday night, agreed to let me go on in his place. Yet even though I got my wish to actually sing on the Opry, the reality of it hadn't really sunk in. I took my place backstage that night, my usual cocky self, acting as if I sang on the Opry every night.

When my time came to sing, none other than Johnny Cash introduced me. "We've got a little girl here from up in East Tennessee," he said. "Her daddy's listening to the radio at home, and she's gonna be in real trouble if she doesn't sing tonight, so let's bring her out here!"

Now the reality hit me. Not only the live audience: I knew very well that the radio broadcast was going out live all over the country. I was in the big time.

I walked up to that mike with the familiar WSM call letters on the little box built around it. *This is actually it*, I thought. For a split second I was a tourist as I pondered the mike, the same one I had seen in so many press photos of the stars I looked up to. I was standing on that same stage in the same place they had stood, where five seconds ago Johnny Cash had stood welcoming me to the stage—me, little Dolly Rebecca Parton from Locust Ridge.

Someone in the audience took a flash picture, and it snapped me out of being a tourist. I wasn't sure I could sing at all. But God had brought me this far and had put something in me that would not be held back. As I heard the band play my introduction, I lifted my head and looked up toward the lights. I smiled at the people in the balcony and then let 'er rip. I sang for God and Mama and Daddy. I sang for everybody who had ever believed in me. Somehow, I believed in me. I guess it showed in my voice.

I was stunned by the way the crowd reacted. I don't think I had ever seen two thousand people in one place before. I know I had never heard a crowd cheer and shout and clap that way. And they were doing it all for me. I got three encores. This time I was prepared for an encore, but not three, not at the Grand Ole Opry. Someone told me later, "You looked like you were out there saying, 'Here I am, this is me.'" I was. Not just to that audience but to the whole world. And I have been doing that same thing ever since.

Dolly Parton

Finding My Wings

*R*each *high, for stars lie hidden in your soul.
Dream deep, for every dream precedes the
goal.*

Pamela Vaull Starr

Like so many other girls, my self-confidence growing
up was almost nonexistent. I doubted my abilities, had
little faith in my potential and questioned my personal
worth. If I achieved good grades, I believed that I was
just lucky. Although I made friends easily, I worried that
once they got to know me, the friendships wouldn't last.
And when things went well, I thought I was just in the
right place at the right time. I even rejected praise and
compliments.

The choices I made reflected my self-image. While in
my teens, I attracted a man with the same low self-
esteem. In spite of his violent temper and an extremely
rocky dating relationship, I decided to marry him. I still
remember my dad whispering to me before walking me
down the aisle, "It's not too late, Sue. You can change your

mind." My family knew what a terrible mistake I was making. Within weeks, I knew it, too.

The physical abuse lasted for several years. I survived serious injuries, was covered with bruises much of the time and had to be hospitalized on numerous occasions. Life became a blur of police sirens, doctors' reports and family court appearances. Yet I continued to go back to the relationship, hoping that things would somehow improve.

After we had our two little girls, there were times when all that got me through the night was having those chubby little arms wrapped around my neck, pudgy cheeks pressed up against mine and precious toddler voices saying, "It's all right, Mommy. Everything will be okay." But I knew that it wasn't going to be okay. I had to make changes—if not for myself, to protect my little girls.

Then something gave me the courage to change. Through work, I was able to attend a series of professional development seminars. In one, a presenter talked about turning dreams into realities. That was hard for me—even to dream about a better future. But something in the message made me listen.

She asked us to consider two powerful questions: "If you could be, do, or have anything in the world, and you knew it would be impossible to fail, what would you choose? And if you could create your ideal life, what would you dare to dream?" In that moment, my life began to change. *I began to dream.*

I imagined having the courage to move the children into an apartment of our own and start over. I pictured a better life for the girls and me. I dreamed about being an international motivational speaker so that I could inspire people the way the seminar leader had inspired me. I saw myself writing my story to encourage others.

So I went on to create a clear visual picture of my new success. I envisioned myself wearing a red business suit, carrying a leather briefcase and getting on an airplane. This was quite a stretch for me, since at the time I couldn't even afford a suit.

Yet I knew that if I was going to dream, it was important to fill in the details for my five senses. So I went to the leather store and modeled a briefcase in front of the mirror. How would it look and feel? What does leather smell like? I tried on some red suits and even found a picture of a woman in a red suit, carrying a briefcase and getting on a plane. I hung the picture up where I could see it every day. It helped to keep the dream alive.

And soon the changes began. I moved with the children to a small apartment. On only $98 a week, we ate a lot of peanut butter and drove an old jalopy. But for the first time, we felt free and safe. I worked hard at my sales career, all the time focusing on my "impossible dream."

Then one day I answered the phone, and the voice on the other end asked me to speak at the company's upcoming annual conference. I accepted, and my speech was a success. This led to a series of promotions, eventually to national sales trainer. I went on to develop my own speaking company and have traveled to many countries around the world. My "impossible dream" has become a reality.

I believe that all success begins with spreading your W.I.N.G.S.—believing in your *worth*, trusting your *insight*, *nurturing* yourself, having a *goal* and devising a personal *strategy*. And then, even impossible dreams become real.

Sue Augustine

Grandma Moses
and Me

I'm too old and it's too late, played over and over in my mind. I was discouraged and exhausted after ending my marriage and my law career at the same time. Despite my intense desire to become a writer, I doubted my ability to succeed as one. Had I wasted years pursuing the wrong goals?

I was at a low point when the voice on the radio began telling the story of Grandma Moses. Ann Mary Moses left home at 13, bore 10 children and worked hard to raise the 5 who survived. Struggling to make a living on poor farms, she managed to provide a bit of beauty for herself by embroidering on canvas.

At 78, her fingers became too stiff to hold a needle. Rather than give in to debility, she went out to the barn and began to paint. On Masonite panels she created brilliantly colored, precisely detailed scenes of country life. For the first two years, these were either given away or sold for a pittance. But at the age of 79, she was "discovered" by the art world—and the rest is history. She went on to produce more than 2,000 paintings, and her book illustrations for *'Twas the Night Before Christmas* were completed in her 100th year!

As I listened to the radio, my mood changed. If Grandma Moses could begin a new career and succeed after 80, my life still had hope after 30. Before the program ended, I charged to my computer to work on the novel I'd nearly abandoned.

It was published eight months later.

Liah Kraft-Kristaine

"We're All Here to Learn"

The future belongs to those who believe in the beauty of their dreams.

Eleanor Roosevelt

"Sixteen," I said. I have forgotten the math question my second-grade teacher, Joyce Cooper, asked that day, but I will never forget my answer. As soon as the number left my mouth, the whole class at Smallwood Elementary School in Norfolk, Virginia, started laughing. I felt like the stupidest person in the world.

Mrs. Cooper fixed them with a stern look. Then she said, "We're all here to learn."

Another time, Mrs. Cooper asked us to write a report about what we hoped to do with our lives. I wrote, "I want to be a teacher like Mrs. Cooper."

She wrote on my report, "You would make an outstanding teacher because you are determined and you try hard." I was to carry those words in my heart for the next 27 years.

After I graduated from high school in 1976, I married a

wonderful man, Ben, a mechanic. Before long, Latonya was born.

We needed every dime just to get by. College—and teaching—was out of the question. I did, however, wind up with a job in a school—as a janitor's assistant. I cleaned 17 classrooms at Larrymore Elementary School each day, including Mrs. Cooper's. She had transferred to Larrymore after Smallwood closed down.

I would tell Mrs. Cooper that I still wanted to teach, and she would repeat the words she had written on my report years earlier. But bills always seemed to get in the way.

Then one day in 1986 I thought of my dream, of how badly I wanted to help children. But to do that I needed to arrive in the mornings as a teacher—not in the afternoons to mop up.

I talked it over with Ben and Latonya, and it was settled: I would enroll at Old Dominion University. For seven years I attended classes in the mornings before work. When I got home from work, I studied. On days I had no classes to attend, I worked as a teaching assistant for Mrs. Cooper.

Sometimes I wondered whether I had the strength to make it. When I got my first failing grade, I talked about quitting. My younger sister Helen refused to hear it. "You want to be a teacher," she said. "If you stop, you'll never reach your dream."

Helen knew about not giving up—she'd been fighting diabetes. When either of us got down, she would say, "You're going to make it. *We're* going to make it."

In 1987, Helen, only 24, died of kidney failure related to diabetes. It was up to me to make it for both of us.

On May 8, 1993, my dream day arrived—graduation. Getting my college degree and state teaching license officially qualified me to be a teacher.

I interviewed with three schools. At Coleman Place Elementary School, principal Jeanne Tomlinson said,

"Your face looks so familiar." She had worked at Larrymore more than 10 years earlier. I had cleaned her room, and she remembered me.

Still, I had no concrete offers. The call came when I had just signed my 18th contract as a janitor's assistant. Coleman Place had a job for me teaching fifth grade.

Not long after I started, something happened that brought the past rushing back. I had written a sentence full of grammatical errors on the blackboard. Then I asked students to come and correct the mistakes.

One girl got halfway through, became confused and stopped. As the other children laughed, tears rolled down her cheeks. I gave her a hug and told her to get a drink of water. Then, remembering Mrs. Cooper, I fixed the rest of the class with a firm look. "We're all here to learn," I said.

Charles Slack, as told by Bessie Pender

A Room of One's Own

Virginia Woolf's *A Room of One's Own* ignited me early on to look for my own special place of peace and solitude. My soul longed for the beauty of some land by a lake—where I could breathe in the scent of pine, listen to the wind in the trees, gaze at an expanse of gray-blue water and follow my dream of writing full-time.

Eventually I followed my heart's desire, leaving a law career to write books, and now the writing was almost paying for the groceries. Book sales and speaking engagements were beginning to grow, too. Spring was in the air, and I was bursting with moxie.

For a year, I had been making payments on a beautiful piece of land on a lake called Oconee. The land had been a miraculous gift—the price was rock-bottom because no one realized that it was lakefront property. I had pitched a tent there and loved sleeping on my own piece of paradise. But now, I was ready to move up. Without savings or the ability to get a mortgage, I was nonetheless determined to build a home, a place of my own.

But how? I knew absolutely no one in the entire county except the real estate agent who had sold me the property.

I didn't know a thing about permits, county laws or building. All I had was an intense thirst to create a nest. I collected names of carpenters from the local hardware store, made some calls and found two who were interested. We haggled about the hourly price—I had no idea how this was supposed to be done.

From my sketched house plan, I estimated the amount of wood needed. Then I held my breath until it arrived, frightened that I had bought too much or too little. I dug holes, poured concrete, sawed wood for the walls and put my new hammer to use for 11 hours straight on the first day. Blisters soon seemed a natural part of the landscape of my hand.

As the building grew to its two-and-a-half story height, my joy was mingled with dread—I had an extreme fear of heights. But when the carpenters needed me on the scaffold for roof beams, I pushed away the nausea and did the work. No one else knew what I had conquered—my fear has never returned.

At the end of five full days, we had put on the roof. Even without walls or windows, it looked like a house that could protect me from at least the rain. So in a rush of exuberance, I moved my sleeping bag in with the lumber and sawdust and sat alone with my awe, my satisfaction and my aching muscles.

Over many months, in every spare moment and with every spare dollar I could find, I completed walls and put in 27 windows, continually learning better ways to do things. Wherever I was, whatever I was doing, I obsessively plotted and planned my next moves. But what a lovely obsession.

Then I faced the big challenges of running water and electricity. Since I still couldn't afford to hire professionals, I bought books, studying them for months before I dared tackle a new project.

My initial work passed the county inspector's critical eye, but I knew that even he couldn't tell if the pipes would withstand the water pressure. The moment finally came to turn the water on. If I had made any big mistakes, I would have a flood inside the house.

After turning on the outside valve, I ran indoors to listen for the dreaded tap-tap of water dripping on wood. I inched my way along every wall. All was quiet. Ecstatic, I turned on the water in every sink and laughed out loud. It was a miracle to have running water for the first time in over a year of building! And I knew every L- and T-connector in the place because I had put in all of them myself.

With writing assignments increasing, I found the cash to have the septic system and drywall installed by professionals. Three days before Easter—one year and eight months from the time I dug the first postholes—I completed installing the last of the kitchen tile. My father and stepmother came for Easter dinner, the first meal cooked in my tiny new oven, and we celebrated the all-important Certificate of Occupancy from the county inspector. As we gazed out onto the sparkling blue lake, with white dogwood petals gracing the view, my heart was so full I couldn't speak.

My dream and I have grown together. And just as I am a work-in-progress, so too is this house. My dream of a simple shelter has become a house with a gazebo and decks, where I can write and create. I have my nest, my place of refuge and solace.

I've learned how to put anything together by seeing the dream in the pieces. How to appreciate the smallest advances and conveniences. How to persevere when no solution is in sight. How to build rather than to blame. This adventure will color the rest of my life, as I dream new dreams and begin the building.

Liah Kraft-Kristaine

Meeting Betty Furness

Opportunities are usually disguised by hard work, so most people don't recognize them.

Ann Landers

It was 1964, the year the tourists shared the famed Atlantic City Boardwalk with the Democratic National Convention.

At the time, I was working as a waitress in a popular steak house, in addition to raising five children and helping my husband with our brand new enterprise—a weekly newspaper. So despite the hoopla and my overflowing tip purse, I was just plain tired and longed for it all to be over.

One evening I approached my next customer without much enthusiasm. She was thinner and daintier than I remembered from her years of opening and closing refrigerator doors on the Westinghouse television commercials in the 1950s, but the cheerful no-nonsense voice was unmistakable. The woman about to dine alone was Betty Furness.

Her warmth and friendliness overcame my awe of waiting on a celebrity. I learned that she had come to Atlantic City to cover the Democratic National Convention from a woman's point of view for her daily radio program. By the time I brought her check, I'd mustered up the courage to ask her for an interview for our little suburban paper. She responded by inviting me to lunch.

As I neared her motel two days later, I was alternately exuberant at my good fortune and nervous at the prospect of interviewing a woman who had once received 1,300 fan letters a week.

I already knew a lot about my subject. A Powers model at 14 and a movie actress at 16, she went on to become a success on the stage. But she was best known for her brilliant career as America's number one saleswoman. The name of Betty Furness was as much a byword of the American household as Westinghouse and its Studio One television program.

That's why, during the interview, her attitude about it all seemed hard to believe—but it was the perfect lead for my story: *"I'll never do another television commercial again as long as I live!"*

She explained to me that when she closed the final refrigerator door on her commercials in 1960, she was determined to carve yet another new career for herself— this time in the news medium. "I know the world is full of information and people wanting that information," she told me. "I want to be part of that."

And yet, even though she worked for CBS News, she'd been told repeatedly that technically she wasn't a news correspondent. "It's what I desperately want to be, but the news media and the public refuse to take my desire to do news broadcasting seriously."

Something about her story connected in my gut. Everyone saw me as "just a waitress," not a writer at all.

"A writer is a person who writes," they said. But when would I ever have the money, time, strength and enough perseverance to make myself who I wanted to be—someone like this woman with four careers behind her that most women would kill for, now seeking yet another for her true fulfillment.

But the real measure of her character, the "dimensions" of this woman's world, emerged in Betty's parting statement. "All my life I've been governed by one philosophy: Do any job you're doing well, and you'll stumble over the right opportunities to do what you truly desire."

In the years that followed that wonderful meeting with Betty, I watched her put her wisdom in action. In only a short time after the convention, her sheer strength of will and positive outlook catapulted her into a new and challenging career as Lyndon Johnson's special assistant for consumer affairs. She went on to become the head of New York State's Consumer Protection Board and the city's Commissioner of Consumer Affairs. When I heard the news, I remembered her philosophy and wished her well.

In later years, I watched her as the first-ever network consumer affairs reporter every night on New York's Channel 5. I laughed in recognition when she discussed manufacturers whose contour sheets didn't fit mattresses. I was glad when she told me what some over-the-counter health remedies really contained. And typical of the reports was one of her last: how to protect yourself from hospitals—all this while she herself was in and out of hospitals for cancer treatments.

Through the years I continued to study her words, which I'd taped across her autographed picture. Amazing things happened in my life as I endeavored to apply those words—ones later reinforced by mythologist Joseph Campbell, who wrote: "Follow your bliss, and doors will open where there were no doors before."

Jobs I'd never anticipated or wanted turned into jobs I loved; unexpected paths took me places I'd never dreamed of. Eventually, stumble by stumble, I believed, began, and went from waitress to dining room manager to hospital public relations director; from newspaper reporter to associate editor of several magazines; from writing consultant to international trainer—and finally, to my dream of professional writer.

The day I saw Betty's obituary, I read that at 76 she'd earned the title of "oldest reporter working on television." As I sat reading about her life and accomplishments, I drifted off to that interview years earlier, when she had shared her secrets of success with me. Little had I realized then the great gift I'd been given by the generous woman who had recognized my frustration that day.

I remembered being swept along by the convention-eers, knowing my life had not been what I truly desired. Yet I had stumbled upon the opportunity to interview her, hadn't I? *Do any job you're doing well, and you'll stumble over the right opportunities to do what you truly desire.*

Yes, over the years we'd separately pursued our dreams and found our opportunities. It had taken talent, vision, a persevering commitment and most important, a strong faith that we could reinvent ourselves.

But it had started at that moment, there on the streets of Atlantic City. Taking a deep breath, I had plunged into the crowd, pushing aside my pyramiding ideas for the piece I would write later that night about Betty Furness. First, I had a job to do well. I had to go feed my share of 14,000 Democrats.

Barbara Haines Howett

8

ON AGING

Grow old along with me!
The best is yet to be . . .

Robert Browning

Keeping Up with Granny . . . and the "Old Guys"

I have always dreaded old age.

I cannot imagine anything worse than being old, maybe infirm, perhaps alone. How awful it must be to have nothing to do all day long but stare at the walls or watch TV.

So last week, when the mayor suggested we all celebrate Senior Citizen Week by cheering up a senior citizen, I was determined to do just that. I would call on my new neighbor, an elderly retired gentleman, recently widowed, who, I presumed, had moved in with his married daughter because he was too old to take care of himself.

I baked a batch of brownies and, without bothering to call (some old people cannot hear the phone), I went off to brighten this old guy's day.

When I rang the doorbell, the "old guy" came to the door dressed in tennis shorts and a polo shirt, looking about as ancient and decrepit as Donny Osmond.

"I'm sorry I can't invite you in," he said when I introduced myself, "but I'm due at the Racquet Club at two. I'm playing in the semifinals today."

"Oh, that's all right," I said. "I baked you some brownies . . ."

"Great!" he interrupted, snatching the box. "Just what I need for bridge club tomorrow! Thanks so much!"

" . . . and just thought we'd visit awhile. But that's okay! I'll just trot across the street and call on Granny Grady." (Now, Granny Grady is not really my grandmother; she is just an old lady who has lived in our neighborhood forever, and everybody calls her "Granny.")

"Don't bother," he said. "Gran's not home: I know, I just called to remind her of our date to go dancing tonight. She may be at the beauty shop. She mentioned at breakfast that she had an appointment for a tint job."

I wished him luck with his tennis game (though I was much more interested in his game with Granny) and bade him good-day.

But I am not easily discouraged. I had set aside that afternoon to call on somebody old, and by golly, I was going to find somebody old to call on!

I called my mother's cousin (age 83); she was in the hospital . . . working in the gift shop.

I called my aunt (age 74); she was on vacation in China.

I called my husband's uncle (age 79). I forgot he was on his honeymoon.

And then I remembered old Sister Margaret, a nun who had been my teacher in grade school. She lived in a retirement home for nuns, and it had been several years since I had seen her. I wondered if the old dear was too senile to remember me.

The old dear wasn't there.

"Whom did you want?" the receptionist had asked when I had inquired if it would be convenient for me to visit.

"Sister Margaret," I had repeated.

"Sister Margaret . . ." mused the receptionist. "Oh! You mean Mercedes! She's away on tour this week."

"Mercedes?" I asked. "On tour?"

"Mercedes is Sister Margaret's stage name," said the receptionist. "When she became an actress, she took the name Mercedes because she had always admired Mercedes McCambridge and because she thought Mercedes sounded more seductive than Margaret."

"She ... uh ... became an actress?" I asked, too stunned to wonder when Sister had learned the meaning of the word "seductive."

"Actually, she's more of a producer-director," the receptionist explained. "A couple of years ago she organized a senior citizens' drama club, and eventually it evolved into a caravan theater. They go all over the state putting on plays. She'll be back Thursday, but she leaves again that evening for Washington, D.C. She's on the White House Commission on Aging, you know."

No, I didn't know, and I can't imagine how she got on such a commission, since she obviously knows nothing about aging!

And I don't want to know about it, either!

I still dread old age, now more than ever. I just don't think I'm up to it.

Teresa Bloomingdale

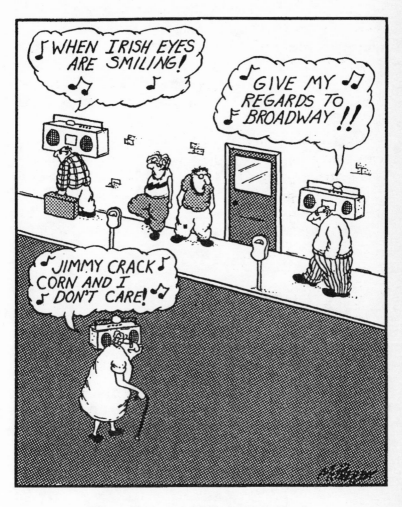

The older generation fights back.

CLOSE TO HOME. ©John McPherson. Reprinted with permission of Universal Press Syndicate.

The Dancin' Grannies

As soon as you feel too old to do a thing, do it!

Margaret Deland

Twelve years ago, when I was 50, I thought, *What will 60 be like? Or 70?* I looked around and saw only one style of being. *It's not fair,* I thought. Young people have so many styles to choose from—they can be yuppies or hippies or what I call regular folks—but older people have just one option, and it doesn't look like much fun. No one seemed to be enjoying themselves. Many people (including me) generally disliked their aging selves. I certainly wasn't happy with the way I looked, and I didn't feel sharp enough to handle everything coming my way. I felt like an insecure teenager all over again!

I decided to do something about it, something practical. I worked on my fitness by joining exercise classes in town. A few years later, my husband and I moved to a retirement community, and I wanted to teach aerobic classes. The community center wouldn't give me a room to teach in, so I had to sneak around and find any available empty room.

One day, the community center staff came to me and asked if I would help with the entertainment for a Hawaiian luau they were putting on. I said yes. (I'm a yes person—I say yes first and think later!) Then I talked five other ladies into dancing with me. *How hard could it be?* I thought. *The hula? Just wiggle your hips!* We performed the hula and a war chant and brought the house down. Someone had a camera and took pictures, then sent them on to our local paper. We got requests for more engagements, which in turn led to more publicity and yet more engagements. Soon we had invitations from all over the country. The Dancin' Grannies were born!

The sad thing was that we met the most resistance from our families and our peers. Older women were disgusted when we performed in leotards and often echoed our children's advice, telling us to "act your age." What did that mean? Being humpy, lumpy and grumpy? No thanks! (Of course, after we were asked to perform at the White House for President and Mrs. Bush and visiting dignitaries, our families changed their tune.)

We often ran into age prejudice. The young in particular assume things about older people that aren't always true. One weekend we were invited to perform at a university in Wisconsin, and it was arranged that we would sleep in the dorms. Well, the students dismantled their bunk beds for us grannies! They must have thought that either we wouldn't be able to get up to the top bunk, or that if we made it up there, we might fall out.

Our performances haven't all been smooth sailing, either. Our first parade was a disaster! I had choreographed a dance number where we started out as old grannies, with hair nets and robes, and then changed into hot grannies—putting on hats and gloves and taking off the robes. Bad Idea! Have you ever tried to change clothes and dance while you're moving with a parade? Plus, as we traveled down the road, the groups who saw the old grannies were not the same people who saw the hot grannies, so the whole point of the dance was lost anyway. Finally, we ended up just changing clothes and then running to catch up. And the audience loved it!

People are amazed at how physically demanding our routines are. We do splits, cartwheels, one-armed push-ups, somersaults and high kicks. Our best cartwheeler is 72 years old.

But I think the real secret of the Dancin' Grannies is our attitude. I was raised extremely poor—no-food poor. If we wanted toys we had to make things up to play with, so I learned early to be very creative. And you know, I think being poor was one of the best things that ever happened to me because I learned to look for treasures.

That's what I'm still doing today—looking for the treasure in growing old. I'm getting better and better. I haven't heard one young person yet say, "I'm just dying to get old—that looks like so much fun!" But it can be. We are pushing the edge of the envelope, living longer in a totally different world. When I was little and visited my grandmother, it was always "Watch out for granny's knickknacks. Don't touch anything. Be quiet." When my grandchildren visit, they like to try and test me, and I say to myself, "I'm not going to let those little twerps beat me!" And oh, we do have fun!

It's true that antiques have to be treated a bit differently, with a little care, but they still have a beauty all their own.

Beverly Gemigniani with Carol Kline

A Romance of the '90s for Those in Their 70s

Age does not protect you from love.
But love, to some extent, protects you from age.

Jeanne Moreau

There he stood, tall and handsome and 71 years old. There I stood, going on 70, and his face went straight to my heart.

We were waiting to see the same doctor at a small Iowa hospital. I sat down right next to him as we both looked at magazines, but I don't think I absorbed a single word I read that day. An hour later, at the local market, I was amazed to find him waiting at the prescription counter as I went up to talk to the pharmacist. I said, "We've got to stop meeting like this." He responded courteously, but I found out later that he hadn't even noticed me the first time!

His name was Bill. As we chatted, I was surprised to discover that this attractive stranger was the father of my granddaughter's kindergarten teacher. His own grandson was also in the class, and the two children had been mysteriously drawn to each other.

Each of us had moved to Iowa from our respective coasts to be close to our children and grandchildren. We had both left unhappy romances behind and were, in a sense, starting over.

The more I learned about this man, the more intrigued I became. He had built his own house with serious environmental consideration. He was an artist and professor of art history. He had been a Conscientious Objector during the war, and in case after case, his values matched mine perfectly.

After a few phone conversations, our two families convened in the town square for a band concert. My daughter insisted that I bake cookies. Apparently they came out pretty good that night.

One day Bill phoned and apologized for not walking me to the door the evening before. I assured him I was a liberated female who didn't need such pampering, and he said, "No, I mean that if I had walked you to the door, I could have given you a good-night kiss."

They say timing is everything. I had been caring for a woman with Alzheimer's disease, and was about to move on. So I was temporarily sharing cramped quarters with my son and his family, planning to find a room to rent somewhere. I stayed with Bill for just a few days when he said, "It would be fun to plan our garden together." That meant our lives were weaving together, and I couldn't have been happier to hear it.

Soon in his sweet, sensitive way, Bill suggested we marry to protect my good name in our closely knit community. I told him I was not concerned with appearances. Then, after a few weeks of what can only be described as domestic bliss, I found myself sitting on his lap one day. He looked at me, smiled, and quietly said, "It would be fun to plan our marriage together." I didn't know my heart could glow like that. How could I possibly say no?

We planned an exquisite June wedding at full moonrise. So many people expressed a desire to witness our union that we put an ad in the local paper in the form of our four grandchildren inviting all to the marriage of their grandparents.

When we exchanged vows, I declared that, "Everything in my life has prepared me for this magical moment." I truly believe that nothing was wasted.

Bill and I came together at a time when both of us had "paid our dues." We'd experienced a lot of pain and a lot of beauty in our lives, and we'd each finally arrived at something like inner peace, self-sufficiency and even self-appreciation.

When I think of our relationship, I think of a passage I once read:

> *I must conquer my loneliness alone.*
> *I must be happy with myself, or I have nothing to offer.*
> *Two halves have little choice but to join;*
> *and yes, they do make a whole.*
> *But two wholes when they coincide . . .*
> *That is beauty. That is love.*

Lillian Darr

Bessie

*F*ew people know how to be old.

La Rochefoucauld

EDITORS' NOTE: The following is an excerpt from *Having Our Say: The Delaney Sisters' First 100 Years,* a memoir of Bessie and Sadie Delaney, two remarkable African-American women who had careers as a dentist and a school teacher before American women had the right to vote. Bessie passed away on September 25, 1995 at the age of 104, and we are honored to include this contribution in her memory.

I'll tell you a story: The house we own is a two-family house, and sometimes the neighbors can hear us through the wall. One time, they had a guest who was up in arms. Just up in arms! She heard these sounds, like laughter, coming from our side, late at night, and she was convinced there were ha'ants. Yes, sir, she thought we were ghosts.

Our neighbor came over the next day and quizzed us down. And I said, "Ain't no ha'ants, it's just the two of us being silly." It hadn't occurred to them that these two old sisters, at our age, would be a-carrying on like that. I guess they think of old folks as people who sit around like old sourpusses. But not us. No, sir! When people ask me how we've lived past 100, I say, "Honey, we never married. We never had husbands to worry us to death!"

I love to laugh. There's a song I just remembered from the 1890s that we colored children used to sing. Sadie and I thought it was hilarious. I hadn't thought of it in, well, about a hundred years! It goes like this:

> *The preacher he went a-hunting*
> *On one Sunday morn*
> *According to his religion*
> *He carried along his gun*
> *He shot one dozen partridges*
> *On his way to the fair*
> *And he got down the road a little further*
> *And spied a big, grizzly bear*
> *Well, the bear stood up in the middle of the road*
> *The preacher dropped to his knees*
> *He was so excited*
> *That he climbed up in a tree!*
> *The parson stayed in that tree*
> *I think it was all night*
> *Then he cast his eyes to the Lord in the sky*
> *And these words said to him*
> *Oh Lord, didn't you deliver Daniel*
> *From the lion's den?*
> *Also brother Jonah*
> *From the belly of the whale,*
> *And when the three Hebrew children*
> *In the fiery furnace sent?*
> *Oh Lord, please me do spare!*
> *But Lord, if you can't help me,*
> *Please don't help that bear!*

Honey, we thought that punch line at the end was just about the funniest thing in the world. Oppressed people have a good sense of humor. Think of the Jews. They know how to laugh, and to laugh at themselves! Well, we colored folks are the same way. We colored folks are suvivors.

There are certain stereotypes that are offensive. Some of them don't worry me, though. For instance, I have always thought that Mammy character in *Gone with the Wind* was mighty funny. And I just loved "Amos 'n' Andy" on the radio. So you see, I have enough confidence in myself that those things did not bother me. I could laugh.

Sadie and I get a kick out of things that happened a long, long time ago. We talk about folks who turned to dust so long ago that we're the only people left on this Earth with any memory of them. We always find ways to celebrate our memories of our family and friends. Why, we still have a birthday party for Papa, even though he's been gone since 1928. We cook his favorite birthday meal, just the way he liked it: chicken and gravy, rice and sweet potatoes, ham, macaroni and cheese, cabbage, cauliflower, broccoli, turnips, and carrots. For dessert we'll have a birthday cake—a pound cake—and ambrosia, made with oranges and fresh coconut.

Generally, we stay away from liquor. Except once in a while, we make Jell-O with wine. What you do is replace some of the water in the recipe with wine. It'll relax you, but you won't get drunk. The truth is, I have never been *drunk* in my life.

One thing Sadie and I do is stay away from doctors as much as possible. And we avoid hospitals because, honey, they'll kill you there. They overtreat you. And when they see how old you are, and that you still have a mind, they treat you like a curiosity: like "Exhibit A" and "Exhibit B." Like, "Hey, nurse, come on over here and looky-here at this old woman, she's in such good shape . . ." Most of the time they don't even treat you like a person, just an object.

One time, some doctor asked Sadie to do a senility test. Of course, she passed. A year later, he asked her to do it again, and she said, "Don't waste your time, doctor." And she answered all the questions from the year before, before he could ask them. And then she said to me, "Come on, Bess, let's get on out of here."

People assume Sadie and I don't have any sense at our age. But we still have all our marbles, yes, sir! I do get tired, physically. But who am I to complain about being tired? God don't ever get tired of putting his sun out every morning, does He? Who am I to complain about being weary?

Funny thing is, some days I feel like a young girl and other days I'm feeling the grave, just a-feeling the grave. That's why it's important that we get all this stuff written down now, because you never know when you'll meet the Lord in the sky.

Bessie Delaney

"Are We Having Fun Yet?"

You don't stop laughing because you grow old;
you grow old because you stop laughing.

Michael Pritchard

Every summer when I was a kid, my family took a two-week vacation at a resort in northern Minnesota. We looked so forward to this annual event that I clearly remember not being able to sleep the night before, and I actually felt my stomach tickle as we drove down the lane of the resort.

The resort was on a lake named Potato. Honest to God, that is still the name of this lake; and no, you don't fish for potatoes. I do, however, remember some rather clever names given to boats: "Sweet Potato," "The Potato Chip" and "Spuds." My dad had visited this lake when he was a kid, and tells us how he was taken in by the sheer beauty of the place and the friendliness of the people. So when he and Mom were married, somehow he convinced her that this was to be their "honeymoon haven." Needless to say, she fell in love, and so our annual vacation saga began.

I don't know when I first met Delores. She was kind of like a relative. You know how it is, you grow up with them, and they are always just sort of around. Delores and her family had a cabin at the edge of the resort and were always actively involved in everyone's vacation. I laugh to myself when I say "actively involved" because Delores was known as the resort's "Activity Director," always drumming up something to do.

I was truly inspired by this woman. You know how every once in a while, you meet someone that touches your soul, as if you were blessed to have known them. Delores was that person for me. She was a petite lady in her early 60s, with tanned skin and a smile that lit up her whole face. Her favorite phrase was, "Are we having fun yet?"

Delores always wore bright colorful outfits with hats and pins or necklaces that her grandchildren had made. She was very sentimental, and it seemed that she always had a tear in her eye over something: a hug from a child, an inspiring song or watching a beautiful sunset. Delores radiated a faith about her. You always felt good about yourself and others when she was around. She found something positive in everyone, and sometimes that's hard to do. I remember her saying, "God made us and is in all of us . . . you just have to search a little harder in some people." Anyone that knew her knew where her priorities were: God, family, friends and loving life. She was actively involved in her church and community, she was a Registered Nurse, and she and her husband, Rich, raised six beautiful children.

Every year over the Fourth of July, Delores planned a big celebration with a boat parade, talent show, raising of the flag, candy hunt for the little kids, volleyball, potluck, fireworks and a campfire sing-along. Oh sure, there were always mumbles and grumbles from people who just wanted to "vacation," but by the end of the day, everyone had participated and, from the smiles and laughter, I would say truly enjoyed themselves.

In the fall of 1991, Delores was diagnosed with cancer. Of course, everyone was devastated by the news. Yet, somehow, I felt that everything was going to be okay. Each year at the lake, we kept thinking that this would be her last "Fourth of July," yet she kept coming back with her colorful red, white and blue hats, planning the celebration once again, and of course asking, "Are we having fun yet?"

By the fall of 1994, Delores was confined to a wheelchair and had to be fed intravenously. We all knew that death was close. One of her daughters told us that Delores had invited her priest over one day and told him, "You know, Father, I have never been scared of dying because I know where I'm going, but I just wasn't ready to go until my family was ready . . . and I think they are ready now." Then she went on to let him know that she really should plan her wake. Her priest had replied, "Sure, Delores, whatever you'd like to do." As the priest started to talk about the formalities of the wake and funeral, Delores interrupted him and said, "No, Father, you don't understand, I want to be there at my wake!"

Two weeks before she passed away, Delores had her "Irish wake," complete with family and friends, Irish toddies, singing, dancing and laughter. Delores sat in the center of the room in her wheelchair, dressed in green with a green Irish hat, and a pin that said, "Kiss me, I'm Irish." What a celebration of life!

A couple of months after Delores' death, her family was sitting around the kitchen table feeling pretty blue and really missing her. Mark, one of Delores' sons, said, "You know, I haven't felt like going to church much anymore. How does anyone really know that there's a God and a heaven?"

Just then, there was a loud BANG! Everyone jumped, and Mark ran over and picked up a plaque that had fallen off the wall. The plaque had been there as long as anyone could remember. It said: "Delores' Kitchen."

Everyone sat there, stunned. Then someone started to giggle, and we all burst out laughing. We could all see Delores, wearing one of her silly old hats, smiling down on us and saying, "Are we having fun yet?"

Kim Miller

$\overline{9}$

HIGHER
WISDOM

Miracles are natural; when they do not occur, something has gone wrong.

Helen Schucman

Asking for Miracles

A number of years ago, author and poet Maya Angelou learned that her only child, Guy, was scheduled for emergency surgery. He had broken his neck in an accident several years earlier, and now complications were arising. So Maya asked for a miracle. Here's how she tells the story.

I went directly to San Francisco to be with Guy. As soon as surgery got under way early the next morning, I drove out to Mission Dolores and I prayed. I had gone there before in a time of trouble—when I was pregnant with Guy and needed help to be allowed to enroll late in a summer school program so that I could finish my high-school education. I had prayed before the statue of Mary then and my prayers were answered. Now I was praying for the life of my son.

When I got back to the hospital six hours later, Guy's doctor was waiting for me. "Success," he said. It was the word I most wanted to hear. I immediately called my sister to tell her the good news. Guy woke up shortly after that. It was late afternoon by then, and everything seemed fine. I stayed around the hospital talking with him and then went back to my hotel.

At midnight the doctor called me. "Ms. Angelou," he said, "we're losing Guy. We've got him back in surgery and we're losing him. You stay there and we'll call you."

Of course, I could not stay in the hotel. I went directly to the hospital, but I didn't go to the surgical floor. Instead, I went to the floor where his room was, and I walked the hall. I walked along past all those half-opened doors, and at times while I was walking I would suddenly feel I was standing on wet sand that was sifting out from under my feet. Then I'd say: "GRAB YOUR LIFE. HOLD ON TO IT. HOLD ON." Loud. For three hours I walked and talked. Then I felt solid.

The doctors came up from surgery. "Ms. Angelou," they said, "we're sorry. He's alive, but he's paralyzed from his neck down." I whispered, "I see. I see." I went down to the intensive care unit and paced in and out waiting for my son to wake up. By 7 A.M. he was awake, and I went in and stood looking down at him. Tubes were coming from everywhere. "Mother," he said, "the thing I most feared has happened. I'm paralyzed."

"It would seem so," I answered.

"I'm your only child," he continued, "and I know you love me, but I refuse to live as a talking head. If there's no chance for recovery, I want to ask you to do something that no one should ever have to ask a mother." The tears were just rolling down his face. "If there's no chance for me to recover, please pull the plug and let me go."

"In that case," I said, "TOTAL RECOVERY, I SEE TOTAL RECOVERY. I SEE YOU WALKING, STANDING, PLAYING BASKETBALL AND SWIMMING. NOW QUIT IT RIGHT NOW. I MEAN IT." That's what I said. Guy started laughing. He said, "Mother, please control yourself. There are some very sick people in here."

The doctors came to talk with me. They said, "Ms. Angelou, Guy has had a blood clot sitting on his spinal cord for eight hours. The cord is so delicate that we don't dare breathe on it. He will never be able to move."

I said, "I'm not asking you, I'm *telling* you. My son will walk out of this hospital and I thank God for it—now!"

One of the doctors started to say, "We all have to . . ."

And I said, "You can't tell me. I'm going somewhere so far, so beyond you, you're not even in it!" And every hour after that I'd say, "TOTAL RECOVERY. I THANK YOU FOR IT. I'M CLAIMING IT FOR THIS BOY. THANK YOU. TOTAL RECOVERY."

The next two days were busy. I called Dolly McPherson, my chosen sister, and she got the whole prayer group at my church together. We had a Jewish sister-friend, and she called people from her synagogue. A Catholic friend called the people she knew in her parish. "Go get everybody, go," I said. "Do what you can do."

The second night, I was lying on a couch in the ICU waiting room when a nurse came in. She said, "Ms. Angelou, Guy's moved his toes." Together we walked to Guy's room. She reached over and pulled the blanket off his feet and Guy moved his toes. I said, "THANK YOU, GOD. DIDN'T I ASK YOU FOR IT AND DIDN'T YOU GIVE IT TO ME. THANK YOU FOR IT. THANK YOU, GOD."

The next morning when I went in to see Guy, he said, "Mama, thank you for your faith. I'll walk out of the hospital." And that is exactly what he did a few months later. I know that prayer changes things. I *know*. I don't question. I *know*.

Maya Angelou
As told to Sherry Ruth Anderson
and Patricia Hopkins

The Wise Woman's Stone

A wise woman who was traveling in the mountains found a precious stone in a stream. The next day she met another traveler who was hungry, and the wise woman opened her bag to share her food. The hungry traveler saw the precious stone in the wise woman's bag, admired it, and asked the wise woman to give it to him. The wise woman did so without hesitation.

The traveler left, rejoicing in his good fortune. He knew the jewel was worth enough to give him security for the rest of his life.

But a few days later he came back, searching for the wise woman. When he found her, he returned the stone and said, "I have been thinking. I know how valuable this stone is, but I give it back to you in the hope that you can give me something much more precious. If you can, give me what you have within you that enabled you to give me the stone."

The Best of Bits & Pieces

Let It Be

I was on the phone the morning of May 13, 1993, when my secretary handed me a note saying that my sister Judy was holding on the other line. I remember thinking it odd that she didn't just leave a message, but I picked up her call with a cheery, "Hi!"

I heard my sister sobbing, as if her heart were broken, as she struggled to gain enough composure to give me her news. A litany of possible tragedies ran through my mind. Had something happened to Aunt Chris or Uncle Leo, our much loved surrogate parents now in their 80s? Judy's husband was out of town. God, I hoped nothing had happened to him! Maybe it wasn't anything that horrible—possibly something had happened with Judy's job.

Nothing could have prepared me for the words Judy finally spoke. "Oh, Sunny, our Tommy was killed in a car wreck this morning."

It couldn't be true. Tommy, my beloved nephew, Judy's only son, was just finishing up his next-to-last semester of graduate studies at the University of Missouri. An athlete, he had chosen to study sports marketing. Tommy's two sisters, Jen and Lisa, had always had a case of hero worship for their big brother. We *all* adored this tall, handsome young man with his easy laugh and gentle nature. Tommy's whole life stretched out before him, and my mind wanted to reject the words I had just heard. I almost asked, "Are you sure?" But even as I thought it, I realized Judy would not have called me otherwise.

My memories of the next few days are a haze of unreality. Lynn, our other sister, and I stayed with Judy and her family during that time, and we all clung to each other for support. I didn't know what hurt worse: the loss of Tommy or seeing my sister act bravely when I knew her world was shattered.

The day we made funeral arrangements was especially hard. No mother should ever have the awful job of selecting a coffin for her child. Judy had so wanted to see her boy one last time, to touch his hand or brush back his hair. But the funeral director had told us she would not be able to see him. Her good-byes would have to be said to that lovingly selected coffin.

That same afternoon, I stood in the front yard of my sister's home and asked my nephew to send us a sign that he was okay . . . to somehow let us know that he had gone on to something even more wonderful than the life we had envisioned for him here. "Sweetheart, can you let us know that you're all right?"

I can't say that I even believed in such things as "signs." But when the heart is in enough pain it will seek comfort in its own way. Tommy's favorite baseball team was the St. Louis Cardinals, so I asked him to send us a cardinal. As I look back on the moment, standing in that yard so full of Tommy's childhood, it was really just a fleeting thought. "Please let us know you're okay. A cardinal will be the sign I'll watch for."

Judy had carefully planned her son's funeral to be a celebration of his life. At my request, she had included Paul

McCartney's beautiful song, "Let It Be." His cousins served
as altar boys and bravely read scripture. The young priest
who said the Mass fought tears throughout the morning.

At one particular moment, as the priest paused to
regain his composure, a bird suddenly began singing
somewhere outside. It was a loud, insistent song that
lasted through the remainder of the service.

It wasn't until later that afternoon, though, that
Tommy's message registered with any of us. A close friend
called us to comment on the beauty of the funeral Mass,
and then said, "When that bird began singing so loudly, I
jerked my head around and saw the most beautiful cardinal sitting in the window of the church!"

I had my sign.

Two weeks later, Paul McCartney came to our city for a
Memorial Day concert. We had already bought tickets for
Tommy and several other family members, and decided to
go ahead with our plans. On the morning of the concert,
as my sister Lynn was dressing for work and listening to
her usual radio station, she heard two disk jockeys talking
about the interview they hoped to get that day with the
famous former Beatle.

Without thinking, she did something completely out of
character—she phoned the radio station and suddenly
found herself telling the story of Tommy and our tragedy,
and of his great love for the Beatles. Could they get the
story to Paul? They couldn't promise, but they'd see what
they could do.

That night, we all settled in for the outdoor concert in
the clear, crisp evening air, cuddled together with our
sweaters and each other for warmth. Over 30,000 had
gathered for the star-billed evening. Paul McCartney
opened with a song that he performed against the back-
drop of an enormous fireworks display. Then, when the
song ended, he waited for silence and said, "Now, ladies

and gentlemen, our next song is for a very special family in our audience. This is for Tommy's family." Then to my two sisters, my nephews and nieces and me, Paul McCartney sang "Let It Be."

As we stood arm in arm, with tears streaming down our faces, candles were lit and other small lights flashed throughout the audience. This was for all of us, especially our Tommy.

K. Lynn Towse with Mary L. Towse

We Are Not Alone

After my husband died suddenly from a heart attack on the tennis court, my world crashed around me. My six children were 10, nine, eight, six, three and 18 months, and I was overwhelmed with the responsibilities of earning a living, caring for the children and just plain keeping my head above water.

I was fortunate to find a wonderful housekeeper to care for the children during the week, but from Friday nights to Monday mornings, the children and I were alone, and frankly I was uneasy. Every creak of the house, every unusual noise, any late-night phone call—all filled me with dread. I felt incredibly alone.

One Friday evening I came home from work to find a big beautiful German shepherd on our doorstep. This wonderful strong animal gave every indication that he intended to enter the house and make it his home. I, however, was wary. Where did this obviously well-cared-for dog come from? Was it safe to let the children play with a strange dog? Even though he seemed gentle, he still was powerful and commanded respect. The children took an instant liking to "German" and begged me to let him in.

I agreed to let him sleep in the basement until the next day, when we could inquire around the neighborhood for his owner. That night I slept peacefully for the first time in many weeks.

The following morning we made phone calls and checked lost-and-found ads for German's owner, but with no results. German, meanwhile, made himself part of the family and good-naturedly put up with hugs, wrestling and playing in the yard. Saturday night he was still with us, so again he was allowed to sleep in the basement.

On Sunday I had planned to take the children on a picnic. Since I thought it best to leave German behind in case his owner came by, we drove off without him. When we stopped to get gas at a local station, we were amazed to see German racing to the gas station after us. He not only raced to the car, he leaped onto the hood and put his nose on the windshield, looking directly into my eyes. No way was he going to be left behind. So into the station wagon he jumped and settled down in the back for the ride to the picnic. He stayed again Sunday.

Monday morning I let him out for a run while the children got ready for school. He didn't come back. As evening came and German didn't appear, we were all disappointed. We were convinced that he had gone home or been found by his owners, and that we would never see him again. We were wrong. The next Friday evening, German was back on our doorstep. Again we took him in, and again he stayed until Monday morning, when our housekeeper arrived.

This pattern repeated itself every weekend for almost 10 months. We grew more and more fond of German and we looked forward to his coming. We stopped thinking about where he belonged—he belonged to us. We took comfort in his strong, warm presence, and we felt safe with him near us. When we saw German come to attention and perk up his ears, and heard that low growl begin deep in his throat, we knew we were protected.

As German became part of the family, he considered it his duty to check every bedroom to be sure each child was snug in bed. When he was satisfied that the last person was tucked in, he took up his position by the front door and remained there until the morning.

Each week, between German's visits, I grew a little stronger, a little braver and more able to cope; every weekend I enjoyed his company. Then one Monday morning we patted his head and let him out for what turned out to be the last time. He never came back. We never saw or heard from German again.

I think of him often. He came when I needed him the most and stayed until I was strong enough to go on alone. Maybe there is a perfectly natural explanation for German's visits to our house—maybe his owner went away on weekends—maybe. I believe German was sent because he was needed, and because no matter how abandoned and alone we feel, somehow, somewhere, someone knows and cares. We are never really alone.

Mary L. Miller

The Hijacking

The flight from New York to Florida began routinely. The flight attendants were busy welcoming passengers, helping them stow their luggage and guiding them to their seats. Since I was first flight attendant, I was going through procedures that were now becoming normal to me after seven months of flying. In my preliminary check of the cabin, I didn't particularly notice the man wearing the black suede cowboy hat and sitting in the third row.

It was an overcast day in 1983. Ten minutes after leaving New York, the plane broke through the clouds. Checking passenger tickets, I came to the man in the cowboy hat and leaned over to ask for his ticket. In a split second of terror, a normal flight turned into a hijacking.

The man jumped up and pinned my left arm behind my back. He whispered in my ear, "I have a gun. Take me to the cockpit." As he jammed the gun into my back, I saw the look of deathly fear in the eyes of the woman who had been sitting next to him, with her little girl. I took a couple of deep breaths and gave the woman and her little girl a reassuring look.

The hijacker was strong; my arm twisted with pain. With the gun pressing into my back, I told the hijacker that the door to the cockpit was pressurized and couldn't be opened for another 15 minutes, when the plane reached an altitude of 30,000 feet. Fortunately, he didn't know there's no such thing as a pressurized cockpit door.

Slowly, I led the hijacker to the back of the plane, as far away from the pilots and passengers as possible. Only a few people knew anything was wrong. Michael, another flight attendant, was conducting beverage service when he caught sight of my face. I don't know what my voice sounded like, but I managed to tell him we had a little problem and that we needed to go to the back of the plane.

It was painfully clear that my own life was not the only one at stake. I thought of the crew, the passengers and their loved ones waiting innocently at the airport. Our survival depended on my absolute composure—I desperately needed a way to calm myself. Trying to ignore the jabbing pressure of the gun in my back, I began to repeat a prayer I learned as a teenager, the Serenity Prayer:

> *God, grant me the serenity*
> *To accept the things I cannot change;*
> *The courage to change the things I can, and*
> *Wisdom to know the difference.*

As I recited the Serenity Prayer, all the procedures I had learned during training to deal with a hijacking came flooding back to me. "Before you officially declare a hijacking, you must see a weapon," they said. I gathered my nerve and told the hijacker I had to see his gun. He pushed it harder into my back. "It's a 32-caliber and if you ask me again, I'll blow a hole right through you."

He then turned to Michael and said, "Call the pilot and tell him we're going to Haiti." Michael complied. After several terrifying moments of silence, the hijacker told

Michael to call the pilot again and tell him to first land the plane in New Jersey, get rid of all the passengers there and then continue to Haiti with just the crew.

This new direction gave me a plan. It was a long shot, but maybe I could convince the hijacker to get off the plane with me in New Jersey. The next 40 minutes felt like a lifetime, but finally, with the gun still pressed to my back, we approached the runway in New Jersey. I turned to the hijacker and said, "You'll never get away with this if we go all the way to Haiti. You'll be arrested and thrown in jail for the rest of your life. If you get off the plane with me here, I'll help you get a car and get away, and no one will ever know."

He said, "No, we're going to Haiti."

The plane landed, and when it finally came to a stop, he turned to me and said, "I've changed my mind—I want it to end."

The silence in the airplane cabin was deafening.

Michael lowered the automatic airstairs, and the hijacker and I walked alone down the stairs and across the airfield. As we walked together, my arm was still twisted behind my back, with the gun pressing into my spine. I wondered where I was going to take him and what I was going to do with him.

Suddenly, out of nowhere, a patrol car appeared on the airfield. The hijacker swung me around in front of him, shielding himself against the police with my body.

That was the moment I was sure I was going to die. I saw my whole family and their reaction to my death. But the Serenity Prayer quickly filled my mind again. "The courage to change the things I can . . ." That's when I felt a peaceful acceptance that became my strength.

I looked back at the plane and watched as the airstairs folded up and the plane slowly pulled away to safety, with my friends and colleagues and all the other passengers on board. I realized with frightening finality that I was on my own.

The hijacker pushed me into the nearest building with him. He waited in the hallway while I entered a nearby office to get him a phone so he could call for a getaway car. When he released my arm for the first time in over an hour, I carefully walked away from him and into the office.

After alerting the tense men inside the office to the danger, I turned and motioned for the hijacker to come in. I calmly explained to him that the two men at the desk were going to help him get a car. When he went to use the phone, it was the first time since the hijacking began that his attention was diverted from me. I knew this was my only chance to escape.

I ran. I thought my heart would pound right out of my chest, but I kept running. It would be impossible to describe the sense of relief I felt when FBI agents and police flooded around me.

Fifteen minutes later they successfully apprehended the hijacker. I was taken immediately to a small room and asked to give a detailed account of the event to the police and the FBI. My heightened memory recalled every nuance of the flight, the crew and the hijacker. They looked at me in amazement and said, "How did you do it? We train people for years to respond like you did. You did everything right."

I simply told them it was a combination of things: good training, good crew and passengers, the ability to handle stress and most of all, faith. As I stood to leave, I looked down and saw underneath the glass top of the table—right where I had been sitting—a copy of the Serenity Prayer.

Name withheld
as told to K. Bernard

Miracle in Toronto

I had absolutely no idea what had driven me from the warmth of a café into this freezing Toronto phone booth. I'd been peacefully drinking a cup of coffee in this strange city when I suddenly had a bizarre but irresistible compulsion to look in the Toronto phone book. Since I knew absolutely no one in Toronto, my compulsion made no sense at all.

I'm British, but I was living in Iowa at the time. I needed a new work visa for the States, so I chose Toronto, since it appeared to be the nearest consulate. And here I was, flipping through the pages of a phone book for apparently no reason. My fingers stopped when I came to McIntyre.

It wasn't an unfamiliar name to me. Twelve years before, the adoption laws had been changed in England, and I'd finally felt ready to trace my birth mother. My search had yielded three facts about her—she had red hair, she was born near Glasgow and her name was Margaret McIntyre Gray. Still, my search had proved fruitless, and I tried my best to put the whole thing out of my mind.

Yet here I was, so many miles from where I started life, staring at several pages of McIntyres. There were so

many names, even under McIntyre, M. I shook myself.
Why was I doing this? I'd been to dozens of cities
throughout the world and had never been reduced to
reading the phone book!

The next thing I knew, the pages were open to Gray. My
eye went down the page and stopped when I found Gray,
M. McIntyre, 85 Lawton Boulevard, Toronto. My brain
seemed to stop at that point—all I could hear was the
sound of my heart. *It's her, it's her,* my heart said. But why
should it be? This was *Canada,* and even if by some bizarre
coincidence she was here, she'd probably be married with
a different name by now. And even if I called, what could
I possibly say? Still, I found myself dialing.

All I could hear on the other end was a strange tone.
Out of order. *I've come too late,* I thought. *That was her, but
she's dead.* I called the repair service. A polite voice
informed me: "Well, there's a contact number, but it's
confidential."

"Look, I know you'll think I'm crazy," I blurted quickly.
"But I think this may be my real mother, whom I've never
known. Can we find out what happened?"

The operator agreed, but when she called the contact
number, a woman informed her that Miss Gray had never
married, so there must be some mistake. Surprised at the
boldness of my own voice, I asked, "Look, would you
mind phoning her again? Tell her that maybe Miss Gray
never married, but I'm here! Tell her the woman I'm looking for was born on July 9, 1914 in Greenoch, Scotland."

That was how I was led to Betty, Margaret McIntyre
Gray's friend. She told me Miss Gray had been ill in the
summer and had left her apartment to live in a residential
home. Oddly enough, although Betty hadn't visited her in
three weeks, she was planning to go that very afternoon.

The next day Betty called. "Well, you're in luck," she
said. "I told Maggie myself and she acknowledged you

immediately. But brace yourself, now—she doesn't want to see you."

I was devastated. But I knew I'd be getting my visa the next day and I'd be flying home by Sunday. Maybe back in the States I'd be able to put the whole thing behind me. Then when I got to the consulate the next day, bureaucratic glitches held up my visa, and I was told I'd have to stay in Toronto for three weeks. Three weeks in the same city with my long-sought mother, and no chance to see her! I didn't know how I could possibly deal with that.

A couple of days later, when the phone rang, I picked it up, dejected. It was Betty, and she could hardly speak for excitement. "Your mother wants to see you Sunday at three o'clock!" she exclaimed. My head felt light with joy and I had to sit down.

When Sunday came, I was too nervous to swallow breakfast. I arrived at the meeting place early, walking around the block twice. And then I saw her . . . a petite, older woman in a green suit, with lots of soft, honey-gold hair. "Hello, dear," she said, the Scots accent strong on her vowels. She grabbed my shoulders and kissed me on the cheek, and then we looked at each other for the first time in 46 years.

We went inside, and she played show-and-tell with an album of photos. I kept looking at her, hoping to see if I had her nose, her hands. But it was her spirit that came through to me that day, an overall feeling I got about her. It didn't take long to realize that I liked her.

Three weeks passed while I waited for my visa, and I saw my mother almost every day. It was a precious time for both of us.

When I finally got my visa, I went to say good-bye. "You know, dear," she said, "I wanted to keep you, I really did, but I just didn't think it would be possible." I assured her everything was okay, and managed to tear myself away to go home. "Remember you're my bubba," she said as I left. At the door, I turned to give her a little wave. She raised her hand in a regal gesture, bidding me adieu.

My mother went into intensive care at Toronto General only three weeks later, fighting a losing battle with pneumonia. I flew back to Toronto to visit her in the hospital. When I entered her room, I immediately noticed a piece of paper lying on her chest. It was the note I had sent her, thanking her for my life. She died the next day.

Sue West

War Story

It was England, 1939. I was 15, and so excited I could hardly keep my mind on my studies. I was too busy preparing to travel from England to France, where I would spend an exciting summer month as an exchange student. The family with whom I would stay had a daughter my age, and she was to come for a month to my home later that summer.

The day of my departure finally arrived, and I was *ready*. My mother came with me on the train ride to London's Victoria Station, where she saw me safely onto the "Channel train" that would take me the rest of the way to Dover. There was never even the suggestion that she would come all the way to the coast with me. I had always been given credit for a lot of common sense, and it didn't occur to anyone that I wouldn't be able to cope with this trip alone.

And so I took the boat across the English Channel, and my big adventure began. My "French family" met me in Paris, where we saw incredible sights—I especially remember the spectacular châteaux along the Loire— before making our way by car to the little village of

Argent-sur-Sauldres, my home for the next four weeks. But I was there only three weeks.

They were a happy three weeks. I was surrounded by many young people, and I still believe that they learned more English from me than I learned French from them. But as time passed, I began to gather that things were not going well on the Continent. There was even talk of war.

Now, war really doesn't fit the thinking of a 15-year-old. One gentleman who spoke a smattering of English took me aside and pointed out the headlines in the paper. Did I want to go home? I felt no urgency. France really wasn't so far away from home; it hadn't taken me *that* long to get over here.

But I began to sense a growing tension in the air and to feel that something was very wrong. My parents had no telephone and there hadn't been a telegram, so I was unsure of how bad things really were.

Then one morning, I woke up and just knew I had to go home. I had a deep intuition that I must get back to England. I immediately talked over my feelings with my host family. They had never given me any outward signs that they wanted me to leave, but once I had made the decision, all plans were put into high gear.

In the wee hours of the following morning, I was on the Paris-bound train, accompanied by my wonderful French mother. The streets of Paris at 6:00 A.M. were eerily deserted . . . *except* for truck after truck filled with French troops. They were headed for the Maginot Line in a brave attempt to ward off the Nazis.

After saying a sad farewell to my dear hostess a week earlier than scheduled, I set out alone on my journey. It was a tense trip home and a long one—three times as long as it should have been—and I was still only 15. I arrived in England at midnight, and there were no buses or taxis to take me the last mile home from the railway station to my house. Although we had sent a telegram, my parents had no idea what time to meet me because transportation schedules had now gone completely haywire. So, almost 24 hours after leaving France, I had to walk the last dark mile alone. No words can describe my feelings the moment I finally rang my doorbell.

Just a few days later, war was declared!

I'll never really know what made me go home when I did. Certainly, the common sense that my parents had instilled in me had stood me in good stead. But I will always believe that it was really my intuition that saved me from spending the war years far from my family in a foreign land.

Maureen Read

Connection

My mother and I are deeply connected by our uncanny ability to silently communicate with each other.

Fourteen years ago, I was living in Evansville, Indiana, 800 miles away from my mother ... my confidante ... my best friend. One morning, while in a quiet state of contemplation, I suddenly felt an urgent need to call Mother and ask if she was all right. At first I hesitated. Since my mother taught fourth grade, calling her at 7:15 A.M. could interrupt her routine and make her late for work. But something compelled me to go ahead and call her. We spoke for three minutes, and she assured me that she was safe and fine.

Later that day, the telephone rang. It was Mother, reporting that my morning phone call had probably saved her life. Had she left the house three minutes earlier, it's likely that she would have been part of a major interstate accident that killed several people and injured many more.

Eight years ago, I discovered that I was pregnant with my first child. The due date was March 15. I told the doctor that was just too soon. The baby's due date had to fall between March 29 and April 3 because that was when my mother had her spring break from teaching. And of course I wanted her with me. The doctor still insisted that the due date was mid-March. I just smiled. Reid arrived on March 30. Mother arrived on March 31.

Six years ago, I was expecting again. The doctor said the due date was toward the end of March. I said it would have to be earlier this time because—you guessed it—Mother's school break was near the beginning of March. The doctor and I both smiled. Breanne made her entry on March 8.

Two-and-a-half years ago, Mother was fighting cancer. Over time, she lost her energy, her appetite, her ability to speak. After a weekend with her in North Carolina, I had to prepare for my flight back to the Midwest. I knelt at Mother's bedside and took her hand. "Mother, if I can, do you want me to come back?" Her eyes widened as she tried to nod.

Two days later, I had a call from my stepfather. My mother was dying. Family members were gathered for last rites. They put me on a speakerphone to hear the service.

That night, I tried my best to send a loving good-bye to Mother over the miles. The next morning, however, the telephone rang: Mother was still alive, but in a coma and expected to die any minute. But she didn't. Not that day, or the next. Or the next. Every morning, I'd get the same call: She could die any minute. But she didn't. And every day, my pain and sadness were compounded.

After four weeks passed, it finally dawned on me: Mother was waiting for me. She had communicated that she wanted me to come back if I could. I hadn't been able to before, but now I could. I made reservations immediately.

By 5:00 that afternoon, I was lying in her bed with my arms around her. She was still in a coma, but I whispered,

"I'm here, Mother. You can let go. Thank you for waiting. You can let go." She died just a few hours later.

I think when a connection is that deep and powerful, it lives forever in a place far beyond words and is indescribably beautiful. For all the agony of my loss, I would not trade the beauty and power of that connection for anything.

Susan B. Wilson

Higher Love

Mom and I were made from the same mold. The same straight brown hair, the same nearsighted brown eyes, the same physique. Mom was my mainstay. Despite all my scholastic achievements and student activities, I was shy and insecure, and she was always there for me. Mom taught social studies at my high school, so all my friends knew and loved her, too.

I was 15 when Mom was diagnosed with lupus and hospitalized for five months. She recovered and went back to teaching, and everything seemed normal. A year later she caught a simple cold that grew into a serious case of pneumonia. Within a week, she was gone. My world abruptly shattered. The door slammed shut on so many possibilities. All the questions I had had about Mom's life and feelings, about my own blossoming womanhood, about seemingly trivial things—like the recipes for our favorite Christmas cookies and Mom's famous lemon meringue pie—now none of those questions would be answered. Mom would never be there, and I was left feeling deeply sad and alone.

My whole personality seemed to change at that point. I had been open and idealistic; now every day I was becoming more bitter and sarcastic. It was as if my heart was armored with grief and guilt. I was haunted by images of my mother's unhappiness. I remembered her sitting on the edge of her bed, weeping, while the rest of the family argued. I remembered so many times when it seemed I could have done more to comfort her.

In my sophomore year of college I learned to meditate and slowly began to emerge from the numbing shell of protection that I had built around myself. Meditation opened the door to dealing with my grief effectively. I'd sit with my eyes closed, and healing tears would flow.

One morning while I was meditating, I remembered caring for Mom when she had returned from the hospital. I had resented the fact that I had to dress her bedsores when I really wanted to hang out with my friends. A flood of guilt and shame welled up in me as I recalled how selfish I'd been.

Just then a thought burst into my head. It was a story Mom had told me about my grandfather, who was stricken with throat cancer when she was eight years old. Before he died, he said to her, "Evalyn, remember this: If anything happens to me and you really need me, call and I will be there for you."

Mom told me that when she was in college, she fell in love with a young man who broke her heart. She felt so distraught that she called out to her father inside herself. She said, "Suddenly, I felt him standing in my dorm room. I felt so loved by him that I knew everything would be all right."

It seemed worth a try, so I cried out to Mom in my mind. "I'm sorry," I sobbed, over and over again. A change came over the room then. Time stood still, and I felt a cloak of peace spread over me. In my heart, I heard my mother say, "All is understood. All is forgiven. There is no need for any regrets." The weight I had carried around all those years seemed released in an instant. I felt a sense of freedom in that moment greater than anything I thought was possible in life.

A few years later, on the eve of my marriage to a wonderful man named Tony, I found myself missing Mom more than I had in years. I longed for her to share the celebration; I needed her wisdom and blessing. Once again I called out to Mom.

The day of my wedding was sunny and glorious—I was soon caught up in the festivities. Afterward, my long-time friend Marilyn approached with a tear-streaked face. She said she wasn't sad; she just needed to talk to me. We made our way to a private corner of the hall.

"Do you know anyone named Forshay?" she asked. "Well, yes," I answered. "My mother's maiden name was Forshar, but it was changed from the French 'Forshay'. Why do you ask?"

Marilyn spoke more quietly then. "During your wedding ceremony, an incredible thing happened. I saw you and Tony surrounded by a light and a presence that was filled with love for you. It was so beautiful it made me cry. And I kept getting that the name Forshay was associated with it."

I was too stunned to say anything. Marilyn continued. "And there was a message that came for you with it. The presence wanted you to know that you will always be loved, to never doubt that, and that this love will always come to you through your friends."

By this time, I, too, was crying, and Marilyn and I held each other. I finally understood that death could not break a connection forged in love. To this day, I will sometimes catch a glimpse of something in the eyes of a friend or loved one, or even my own eyes in the mirror, and I know my mother is still here, loving me.

Suzanne Thomas Lawlor

I Wonder Why Things Are
the Way They Are

During my junior year in high school, Mr. Reynolds, my English teacher, handed each student a list of thoughts or statements written by other students, then gave us a creative writing assignment based on one of those thoughts. At 17, I was beginning to wonder about many things, so I chose the statement, "I wonder why things are the way they are?"

That night, I wrote down in the form of a story all the questions that puzzled me about life. I realized that many of them were hard to answer, and perhaps others could not be answered at all. When I turned in my paper, I was afraid that I might fail the assignment because I had not answered the question, "I wonder why things are the way they are?" I had no answers. I had only written questions.

The next day Mr. Reynolds called me to the front of the class and asked me to read my story for the other students. He handed me the paper and sat down in the back of the room. The class became quiet as I began to read my story:

Mommie, Daddy . . . Why?

Mommie, why are the roses red? Mommie, why is the grass green and the sky blue? Why does a spider have a web and not a house? Daddy, why can't I play in your toolbox? Teacher, why do I have to read?

Mother, why can't I wear lipstick to the dance? Daddy, why can't I stay out until 12:00? The other kids are. Mother, why do you hate me? Daddy, why don't the boys like me? Why do I have to be so skinny? Why do I have to have braces and wear glasses? Why do I have to be 16?

Mom, why do I have to graduate? Dad, why do I have to grow up? Mom, Dad, why do I have to leave?

Mom, why don't you write more often? Dad, why do I miss my old friends? Dad, why do you love me so much? Dad, why do you spoil me? Your little girl is growing up. Mom, why don't you visit? Mom, why is it hard to make new friends? Dad, why do I miss being at home?

Dad, why does my heart skip a beat when he looks in my eyes? Mom, why do my legs tremble when I hear his voice? Mother, why is being "in love" the greatest feeling in the world?

Daddy, why don't you like to be called "Gramps"? Mother, why do my baby's tiny fingers cling so tightly to mine?

Mother, why do they have to grow up? Daddy, why do they have to leave? Why do I have to be called "Grannie"?

Mommie, Daddy, why did you have to leave me? I need you.

Why did my youth slip past me? Why does my face show every smile that I have ever given to a friend or a stranger? Why does my hair glisten a shiny silver?

Why do my hands quiver when I bend to pick a flower?
Why, God, are the roses red?

At the conclusion of my story, my eyes locked with Mr. Reynolds's eyes, and I saw a tear slowly sliding down his cheek. It was then that I realized that life is not always based on the answers we receive, but also on the questions that we ask.

Christy Carter Koski

10

ACROSS THE GENERATIONS

I am the woman who holds up the sky.
The rainbow runs through my eyes.
The sun makes a path to my womb.
My thoughts are in the shapes of clouds.
But my words are yet to come.

Ute poem

THE FAMILY CIRCUS

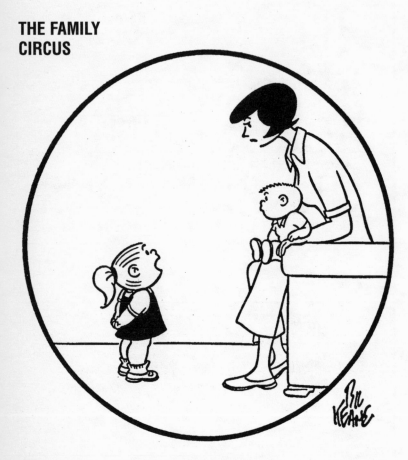

"Was there an older generation when you were little, Mommy?"

Reprinted with special permission of King Features Syndicate.

On Giving Birth

When a child is born, so are grandmothers.

Judith Levy

There is something to be said about leaving a piece of yourself behind in the form of children. Twenty-seven years ago I looked upon my daughter for the first time as she was laid upon my belly, her umbilical cord still attached to me. Her little eyes seemed endless as she looked at me. I witnessed a piece of myself lying there, and yet she was so curiously and wondrously unique.

Today I stand next to her, wiping her face and reminding her to focus on the birthing movements of her own body instead of on pain and fear. She has always been utterly terrified of pain. Yet here she is . . . refusing all drugs . . . living her determination to birth her baby as nature would have it, as did the endless stream of her great-grandmothers before her.

Centuries of pushing, preparing, sighing—and then my daughter's daughter is placed across her mother's breast, staring into her mother's eyes. The Great Mystery is blessing me again, letting me see my granddaughter, the piece of myself who will step into the future and in turn mold her own child, my great-grandchild.

Kay Cordell Whitaker

A Doll for Great-Grandmother

When my grandfather died, my 83-year-old grand-mother, once so full of life, slowly began to fade. No longer able to manage a home of her own, she moved in with my mother, where she was visited often by other members of her large, loving family (two children, eight grandchildren, 22 great-grandchildren and two great-great-grandchildren). Although she still had her good days, it was often hard to arouse her interest.

But one chilly December afternoon three years ago, my daughter Meagan, then eight, and I were settling in for a long visit with "GG," as the family calls her, when she noticed that Meagan was carrying her favorite doll.

"I, too, had a special doll when I was a little girl," she told a wide-eyed Meagan. "I got it one Christmas when I was about your age. I lived in an old farmhouse in Maine, with Mom, Dad and my four sisters, and the very first gift I opened that Christmas was the most beautiful doll you'd ever want to see.

"She had an exquisite, hand-painted porcelain face, and her long brown hair was pulled back with a big pink bow. Her eyes were blue as blue could be, and they opened and closed. I remember she had a body of kidskin, and her arms and legs bent at the joints."

GG's voice dropped low, taking on an almost reverent tone. "My doll was dressed in a dainty pink gown, trimmed with fine lace. But what I especially remember was her petticoat. It was fine batiste, trimmed with rows and rows of delicate lace. And the tiny buttons on her boots were real. . . . Getting such a fine doll was like a miracle for a little farm girl like me—my parents must have had to sacrifice so much to afford it. But how happy I was that morning!"

GG's eyes filled and her voice shook with emotion as she recalled that Christmas of long ago. "I played with my doll all morning long. She was such a beautiful doll. . . . And then it happened. My mother called us to the dining room for Christmas dinner and I laid my new doll down, ever so gently, on the hall table. But as I went to join the family at the table, I heard a loud crash.

"I hardly had to turn around—I knew it was my precious doll. I just knew it. And it was. Her lace petticoat had hung down from the table just enough for my baby sister to reach up and pull on it. When I ran in from the dining room, there lay my beautiful doll on the floor, her face smashed into a dozen pieces. I can still see my mother trying to put my poor dolly together again. But it couldn't be done. She was gone forever."

A few years later, GG's baby sister was also gone, she told Meagan, a victim of pneumonia. Now the tears in her eyes spilled over—tears, I knew, not only for a lost doll and a lost sister, but for a lost time.

Subdued for the rest of the visit, Meagan was no sooner in the car going home than she exclaimed, "Mom, I have a great idea! Let's get GG a new doll for Christmas, one exactly like the doll that got broken. Then she won't cry when she thinks about it."

My heart filled with pride as I listened to my compassionate little daughter. But where would we find a doll to match GG's fond memories?

Where there's a will, as they say, there's a way. When I told my best friends, Liz and Chris, about my problem, Liz put me in touch with a local dollmaker who made doll heads, hands and feet of a ceramic that closely resembled the old porcelain ones. From her I commissioned a doll head in the style of three-quarters of a century ago—making sure to specify "big blue eyes that opened and closed," and hands and feet. From a doll supply house I ordered a long brown wig and a kidskin body, and Meagan and I shopped for fabric, lace and ribbon to duplicate the outfit GG had so lovingly described. Liz, who had some experience with a hot-glue gun, volunteered to put the doll together, and as the last days before Christmas raced by, Chris helped me make the doll's outfit, complete with lacy petticoat. And while Liz, Chris and I searched for doll "boots with real buttons," Meagan wrote and illustrated the story of the lost doll.

Finally, our creation was finished. To our eyes it was perfect. But, of course, there was no way it could be *exactly* like the doll GG had loved so much and lost. Would she think it looked anything like it?

On Christmas Eve, Meagan and I carried our gaily wrapped gift to GG, where she sat surrounded by children, parents, aunts, uncles, cousins. "It's for you," Meagan said, "but first you have to read the story that goes with it."

"Read it out loud," one of the other children demanded. GG no sooner got through the first page than her voice cracked and she was unable to go on, but Meagan took over where she left off. Then it was time to open her present.

I'll never forget the look on GG's face as she lifted the doll and held it to her chest. Once again her tears fell, but this time they were tears of joy. Cradling the doll in her frail arms, she repeated over and over again, "She's exactly like my old doll, exactly like her."

And perhaps she *wasn't* saying that just to be kind. Perhaps however impossible it seemed, we *had* managed to produce a close facsimile of the doll she remembered. But as I watched my eight-year-old daughter and her great-grandmother examining the doll together, I thought of a likelier explanation. What GG really recognized, perhaps, was the love that inspired the gift. And love, wherever it comes from, always looks the same.

Jacqueline Hickey

Walking One Another Home

"If we let Mom stay alone in the house any longer, it will be neglect."

My brother's words to me on the phone set in motion an immediate sequence of events that include helping our mother move from the little house where she has lived for nearly 60 years into a retirement home apartment a hundred miles away. We will have a week to get the house packed up. In my mind's eye I see her standing helplessly in her yellow kitchen, shoulders drooped, sensing something "bad" is about to happen, but not always remembering what. I cannot bear the thought of her last seven long days in that house—alone and facing a heart-wrenching move from her precious roots.

I teach my classes the next day and catch a red-eye special home to help her.

The seven days that follow are bittersweet ones: some of the richest days of my life, but some of the most challenging and poignant. Mom's state of mind is immediately apparent. Over the phone she had told me she'd begun to pack, but when I arrive, only two cardboard boxes stand open in the back bedroom. At the bottom of one box lie two little lace doilies she crocheted before she and Dad got married. The other contains three rolls of toilet paper— nothing more. This is the extent of her "packing"; the rest is too overwhelming. "I just don't know where to start, Rita." Already my heart is weeping with her.

We do not start with packing. In fact, the whole week I am there, we do not take down a single picture or upset the orderliness of the house in any way. (My sisters' orders: "You be the advance team, Rita. Just be with her in the grieving and in the good-byes. When *we* get there, we'll pack. Okay?")

I try to think of what might lift Mom's spirits: maybe we can walk a bit by the lake—that's sure to do it. Some of my earliest and sharpest memories of my mother are of her walking, everywhere, for the family owned no car.

What a confident, joyful walker she was! One remark- ably vivid picture is engraved on my nine-year-old mind: It is a hot August day. Mom is striding briskly along the lake across from our house—toward the hospital on the other side—on her way to give birth to my sister Mary. On her way to give birth? Striding? Briskly? Yes. Dad could scarcely keep up with her.

In a way, walking has always been a prime measure of Mom's state of well-being. Walking helps feed and create a positive sense of herself, gives her a feeling of aliveness, of vitality.

In later years, when all her kids are launched, walking around that little lake across from our house becomes a daily treat for Mom—once she has a car and doesn't have to walk everywhere else. It is also a favorite ritual of ours when I come to visit. In the past three or four years, how- ever, with her feet swollen and painful, Mom has not been up to it, much to her great dismay. Nevertheless, before I start out, I always ask anyway, "Are you able to go walk- ing today, Mom?"

On my first day back, much to my surprise—as if she's been waiting—she answers, "I sure am!" The lake is maybe a third of a mile around. We traipse around it three times, without a rest, pausing at each completed round to see if it is time to head home. "Let's keep going!" she grins. ("See, I can still do *this!*") We are both amazed and delighted at her newfound stamina. And she is very proud.

But the following days, she can scarcely walk at all, and certainly not around the lake; even getting in and out of the car becomes a strain. "I must have overdone it that first day, Rita." Still, each day when I am ready to go walking, I invite her to join me, just in case she's up to it again. Both of us are disappointed when she is unable to take even a leisurely stroll.

During those seven days, Mom and I laugh a lot, cry a little. We keep life pretty normal. Some mornings we go to Mass. Sometimes we invite favorite cronies out to lunch. At any time of the day or night, we find ourselves plunked down in the easy chairs in the living room, just gazing for hours at our favorite sight: the lake and the trees across from our house. How she loves that lake! We all do. We watch some television—the news, especially the weather, Lawrence Welk, *Wheel of Fortune.*

Each day the magic hour of five o'clock ushers in "happy hour." At 4:55, Mom begins arranging hors d'oeuvres while I fix drinks. And we always clink our glasses in a toast to signal that "happy hour" has officially begun. (More than once that week, words for the toast stick in my throat.) After happy hour, we fix dinner together. Pop popcorn later. Maybe play some pinochle. All the while, a cloud hangs over these common ordinary things that we've enjoyed through the years.

Mom's mini-strokes some weeks before have left her unable to drive, so we run errands she's not been able to do alone—go to the bank, to the grocery store, to Kmart for denture tablets and other supplies. I drive her to get her hair permed for the last time by the woman who has done it for 35 years, to get her taxes figured by the same accountant who has performed that task for the Bresnahans since the early 1930s. Back at the house, we find ourselves just sitting and looking at that lake again, sometimes quietly, at other times reminiscing.

Certain aspects of the lake always intrigue her:

"See how the water glistens, just like diamonds."

"The waves are really high today, aren't they, Rita!"

"Isn't the fountain pretty?"

"Look at all the people walking today. Do you see that one in the funny red hat?"

Too soon, my time with her comes to an end. On my last day home, the last day I will ever spend in this little house, I rise early so as to get some exercise before leaving for the airport. Mom is awake but still in bed, and to my usual invite to go for a walk, she answers, with sadness in her voice, "No, my legs are hurting me too much. You go ahead."

My heart is heavy as I step out into the chill—a foggy Illinois morning, with visibility perhaps 100 yards or so. Setting off briskly, I spot a few other hardy souls, mere shapes in the mist, out for their morning constitutional. I circle the lake three or four times, then as I am rounding the curve that puts me in front of our little house, I discern a lone figure wearing a long garment, approaching slowly through the mist. As the figure draws closer, I realize it is my mother. She raises her hand in a wave, and I hurry to meet her, shouting, "Mom!" A long brown raincoat covers her flimsy nightgown.

"I just had to come meet you, Rita. Are you going around again?"

"Oh, I don't know, Mom. Do *you* feel like it?"

She is quiet for a moment, torn, it seems, by an inner struggle—between her unflagging spirit that has navigated that lake for almost 60 years and longs to walk it one last time, and every bone and muscle in legs that can no longer carry her and that shout, "No way!" The struggle registers in her face, she slowly shakes her head, looks down into the lake with a great sadness and murmurs haltingly, "Oh—Rita—let's—just—walk—one another home."

We turn around, and arm in arm, step by step, Mom and I begin shuffling the five minutes back toward our little house. It's our last walk together here—we know it in our bones. Tears start, for both of us. I can feel her chest heaving, there where our arms are interlocked. As for myself, 58 years of memories are crowding in and streaming down my cheeks. We hold tightly onto one another's arm.

The little house welcomes us back into the shelter of its warmth. It feels more like holy ground to me than it ever has before, rich with the fullness of life that has been lived here. Holy ground where, as a little girl, I learned not only how to walk, but how to "walk with one another." Waves of gratefulness wash over me for all my parents taught me here, and for my mother's walking . . . especially for her walking . . .

I help Mom out of the damp raincoat and into her warm blue bathrobe with the lacy cuffs. Shuddering and shivering as she ties the robe, she goes straight to the stove and puts the teakettle on as she's done every morning for 60 years. "C'mon, Rita. Let's sit down and have a cup of tea."

Rita Bresnahan

The Making of a Woman

I watched with my dad as my mother came down the stairs. First appeared the tips of her red satin high heels, followed by smooth, creamy legs. The hem of her gray, watered-silk Chanel floated into view like a fog. The skirt funneled upward to a cinched waist, which began at once to reach outward again to claim a pair of proud, under-wired breasts, pressing against a red satin wrap that framed her bare shoulders and tucked in behind her elbows. She was the epitome of '60s chic. Her scent reached us . . . heady, delicious.

I turned toward my father to see how he liked it and was riveted by a new expression on his face. He stared up at this creature-no-longer-his-wife with a glowing gaze that seemed to impale her like a butterfly on a pin. She stopped, midstep. A slightly startled smile touched her lips. "Well," she murmured, "how do I look?"

"Come here, you," he said—commanded.

I stared at these two people who had once been my parents. They seemed to share some secret that, strange as it seemed, obviously had nothing to do with me. I felt a sudden urge to wedge myself in between them. I saw him put her evening coat over her shoulders. He bent down and whispered something into her hair and she tilted back her head. A secret dawned in her eyes. Like the shutter of a camera, my mind captured that instant. It remained with me long after the door had closed behind them.

The next day I sat in my father's chair waiting for him to come home. I wore my mother's Chanel, the cinch belt pulled well past the last notch. I had found that when I sucked in my stomach and raised my ribcage, I gave a perfect impression of having breasts. I waited, my bare legs stretched in front of me like a model's. I noticed the lipstick smear from when the tube had dropped from my hand, bounced off the bathroom counter and slalomed down the skirt. I hid it in a fold of fabric. Then I heard the key in the lock. Quickly I lifted my chest.

He stopped when he saw me, about to say hello as usual, but registering something different. I could practically see his workday drop from his mind like a dusty backpack as he took in the dress, the made-up face, the pose. His eyes softened, and then his face adopted a smile of pure Desi Arnaz charm. "Well!" he said. "Is this my lucky day? Let's have a look at you." I got off the chair and rustled toward him, stepping carefully. His amused eyes dropped to the red streak across the skirt, and his expression changed. He looked at me sharply. I stopped, for the first time realizing what I'd done: my mother's favorite dress, impossibly expensive, a Christmas gift from Dad. We stared at each other, his eyes seemed to knife right through me . . .

Suddenly he crouched down and looked into my face. I saw the crinkles around his eyes, little white untanned rays, and the lank, brown hair with the blond layer on top. I saw my own skinny little body engulfed in this ocean of watered silk. Then I heard him whisper to me, "You're growing up so fast, you know that? Someday I'm gonna turn around and you'll be the toast of the town. Your old Dad won't be able to fight his way through the boys. Will he?"

All at once he picked me up and held me in a gigantic bear hug. My mother's shoes flew from my dangling feet, landing noiselessly somewhere on the carpet. He squeezed the breath out of me, five o'clock shadow dug into my neck, drawing a muffled scream of laughter before he gently put me back down. He crouched again. "Don't grow up too fast, you," he ordered. He tapped my flat, unremarkable nose.

And for the first time he didn't call it "the freckle farm."

Doni Tamblyn

Tribute to Dad

My father died three weeks after his 80th birthday. No one read about it in the headlines since he'd never invented anything to speak of or lit up the big screen or amassed a huge fortune. His most outstanding achievement was that he was a nice guy. But that seldom makes the headlines. "Harold Halperin, Nice Guy, Dies at Age 80."

For most of his adult life he owned a corner drugstore with his brother-in-law. It was the old-fashioned kind of store with friendly service, a soda fountain and a gumball machine where the gum still cost a penny and you could even get a "winner" to trade in for a candy bar. Although his customers could have bought their prescriptions cheaper at the chain across the street, they came to my dad's because his "Hello, Mr. Jones!" did more to heal than any of the drugs.

When he retired at the age of 70, my dad started a second career working for the Hershey Company, stocking candy racks at the local 7-Eleven's and White Hen Pantries. Although he was supposed to throw away the outdated candy bars, one of his greatest pleasures in life was to share them with the neighborhood kids or bring them to the local soup kitchen for the homeless to enjoy. Everyone called him the Candyman.

His entire illness, from the time he was diagnosed with pancreatic cancer to the time he died, was less than four months. Those four months were a gift to him and to us— not long enough for him to suffer a great deal, but long enough for all of us to say our good-byes and to feel complete. It was also a time for me to notice not only who he was but also the way my father gave us his love. I had never taken the time to notice before.

I delivered his eulogy:

> *Yesterday morning, on the Sabbath, my beautiful father died. When thinking about the words to say at his funeral, I thought, "What tribute can you pay a man whose whole life was a tribute? A tribute to goodness, kindness, caring and generosity. There's really no need for words because my dad's life spoke loud and clear enough."*
>
> *We all know who Harold Halperin was. He was everyone's favorite friend. He was everyone's favorite neighbor. He was everyone's favorite uncle. He was everyone's favorite employer. He was everyone's favorite employee. He didn't have an enemy in the world. I don't think there was anyone who knew him that didn't love him. He was a gentleman and a gentle man.*
>
> *Not that he was perfect—no human being is. But in my life, even in the most trying times for him—and there were a few where I really stretched the guy—I never felt for even a moment that he wasn't there for me with all his heart and all his love.*
>
> *We're all going to miss him. I'm going to miss him because he was the only one who told me on a regular basis that I was so beautiful that I should have been a movie star—and really believed it.*

The kids will miss him because there was never a more loving grandpa. I wish you could have seen the way he played with his grandchildren. The love in his eyes, the way he adored them—and how they loved him! It was always, "Papa, look at me," "Papa, come here," "Papa, watch," "Papa, play with me!" And there he was, down on the floor with them, not caring how difficult it was to get back up again.

And my mom—what can I say about their love? For 47 years those two were completely devoted to each other. My husband and Mom were talking yesterday and Mom said, "If only you and Debbie could have a marriage like Harold and I had. In 47 years, we never went to bed angry." To which my husband replied, "Ceil, I think we blew it already."

One of my most vivid memories of childhood was when my dad would come home from work at 6:30 for dinner. My brother and I would hear him ring the bell— our private joke was that he'd ring it over and over until we got there. We'd be upstairs doing our homework or watching TV and we'd yell to each other, "Daddy's home, Daddy's home!" Then we'd race downstairs and open the door and he'd always say, "What took you so long?" It was the highlight of our day when Dad came home.

A second vivid memory was the dinner ritual he had. When we'd be sitting at the table, Daddy would reach over and put his hand on Mom's arm and say, "Do you two know that you have the most wonderful mother in the world?" He'd say that every night.

And my mom and dad lived his final weeks as they lived the rest of their lives together—my mother loving him and taking care of her darling, precious husband's every need, 24 hours a day. Doing everything that was humanly possible so that he could die with dignity in his own bed without suffering.

And my dad, with days, even hours, left in his life, was still wanting to make sure everything was taken care of for his wife and family. A few days ago Dad was so weak he could hardly talk, and I was telling him how much I loved him and what a great dad he'd been and how lucky Larry and I were to have him for our father. I was going on and on, pouring my heart out to him, and finally I just said, "I love you so much, Daddy." At which point he whispered something back to me. At first I couldn't hear him, so I put my ear close to him and said, "What did you say?" He mustered all his strength and repeated, "Be sure to get the brakes on the Oldsmobile fixed. I don't want your mother driving without good brakes."

There's a lot of press these days about how there are no heroes or great men for our children to look up to. My dad might not have won a Nobel prize, but if you want an example of a great man, you don't have to look further than Harold Halperin.

Mom and I will never forget how sweet and peaceful you looked on the morning you died, with the sun pouring in the eastern window, illuminating your silver hair as if a thousand angels were dancing around you.

And we'll never forget that even though the neighbor's dog barked and barked every night for all the months you were sick, he didn't make a peep the night you died, but sat as still as stone hour after hour, staring up at your bedroom window as if he were the official guard at heaven's gate.

So we love you, Daddy. You were as beautiful in death as you were in life. We'll miss you but will never forget who you were, and we'll always talk about you and tell our children and our grandchildren about their grandpa who, although he tried to fix major appliances with string and Scotch tape, was in our eyes one of the greatest men who ever lived.

Now go and be with God and be in peace.

We love you.

Debra Halperin Poneman

Memories of a Childhood Past

Most of all the other beautiful things in life come by twos and threes, by dozens and hundreds. Plenty of roses, stars, sunsets, rainbows, brothers and sisters, aunts and cousins, but only one mother in the whole world.

Kate Douglas Wiggin

She sits passively in front of the television. It does not seem to matter what program is on, as long as she does not have to get up to change the channel. Walking, like everything else, has become difficult for her. She needs assistance to get dressed, to eat and to bathe. It is not because her body has become old and crippled—she is only 48—but her mind has. She has Alzheimer's disease. She is my mother.

Sometimes it seems as if no time has passed since I was a child and we went on nature walks together. The natural environment was one of my mother's passions. She would take me to the beach to explore the tide pools. We would jump from one rock to the next, carefully trying to avoid the waves crashing only a few feet away. She would point out the purple-spiked sea urchins and brightly colored sea stars. I can still feel the fine mist of sea water on my face and smell the salty air. She also liked to take me on hikes in the redwoods after the rain. We would search for banana slugs, whose bright yellow color glowed like little night lights in the darkness of the woods. We could smell the dampness of the leaves as we walked among those giant skyscrapers and lost ourselves in the majesty of that enchanted place.

Deeply affected by the political activism of the 1960s, my mother believed in fighting for what was right and protesting what was not. She was not a radical; she was just concerned about the world and the people in it. I can remember going on a peace march with her when I was about 10. It was a silent nighttime walk through downtown. Each one of us held a candle that illuminated the night and symbolized our hope to bring light to the world through our silent message.

Education was another thing that was important to my mother. She was a teacher who had put herself through graduate school when I was in elementary school. I still do not know how she did it. Even in the midst of her studies, I cannot remember a time when I felt that she was not there for me. Because she was an educator herself, she did a lot of research before choosing a kindergarten for me. While most parents simply settle on the school closest to their home, my mother took me to observe several schools before she found one that she was satisfied with.

Now I often look at my own daughter and see my mother. I see my mother's average brown hair beautifully woven with golden blonde strands and auburn highlights. I see her chin that juts out slightly from her narrow face and the extra crease in the fold of one of her eyelids—

they are the same features my mother must have seen when she looked at me and saw herself.

Lately I have noticed that I surround myself with things that remind me of her. Every time I drink a cup of Sleepytime tea, the soothing smell reminds me of all the sleepless nights my mother spent holding me when I was ill. When I get dressed in the morning, the herbal-scented lotion and sweet, fruity hairspray I use are the same as those my mother used to buy. When I listen to the political twang of a Joan Baez song or the rhythmic pulse as Jimmy Cliff sings a reggae chant, I can hear my mother's voice. There is rarely a day that goes by without my hearing, smelling, tasting or seeing something that brings back memories. These things are comforting and allow me to escape to my childhood, when my mother was still the way I remember her.

This disease has quickly stolen the woman I once knew. She had always taken such an active role in life, and now she sits so still. I read a poem once, "To My Alzheimer's Mother," that puts this idea to words beautifully:

> *Sweet Mother with your bright blue eyes*
> *Seeing you empty—how my heart cries*

My mother may not remember all that she did to impact my life, but I have not forgotten. The hardest thing for me is learning to love the mother I have now while still enjoying the memories of who she used to be. I pray for her almost every night, but my prayers have changed. I used to pray, "Lord, let them find a cure." Now I simply ask, "Lord, just let her be happy in her own world, as she made me happy in mine." Sometimes, almost hoping that she will somehow hear me, I whisper, "I love you, Mom. I miss you."

Sasha Williams

Threads That Bind

Love is the emblem of eternity; it confounds all notion of time.

Anna Louise de Staël

The quilt was obviously very old. Many of the silk fabrics had almost disintegrated with time, but still it was beautiful. It was a variation of a Log Cabin, a small square in one corner with logs on only two of the sides. Yes, the fabrics were worn and fading, but it had evidently been well cared for over the years.

The quilt teacher held the quilt up for all to see. "This is a type of Log Cabin quilt quite popular in the mid-1800s. This particular one must have been made by someone who had access to many fabrics because of the variety used in the quilt. After I bought it, I noticed it had originally been larger. Someone had cut it in half." Everyone in the class moaned. Who could have possibly ever cut into such an exquisite quilt?

A wagon train headed west; it was 1852 . . .

Katherine reflected on the events of the past three

years as she pulled the quilt up around herself and her sister, Lucy. Today had been a happy day; Katherine and Lucy had celebrated their common birthday. Katherine had just turned 13 and Lucy three. Katherine had been exactly 10 years old when her sister was born. How happy she had been to finally have a little sister! All her friends had very large families, and Katherine had wanted a brother or sister for a long time. Finally her wish had come true: She had a sister, a sister born on her own birthday. The family members were all so happy. It seemed as if nothing could ever go wrong.

Tragedy struck, however, when Lucy was a year-and-a-half old. Their mother died. Soon after that, Father decided that the little family should move west. Everything was sold, given away or packed into a wagon, and they headed out. In spite of her joy over the birthday celebration earlier in the day, Katherine shivered and pulled the precious quilt closer around them. The quilt was all she had to remind her of mother and home.

Lucy broke into Katherine's reverie: "Tell me a story," she begged. "Tell me a story from the quilt."

Katherine smiled. Every night was the same. Lucy loved the stories from the quilt, and Katherine loved telling them. It helped her remember happier days.

"Which one?" she asked.

Lucy moved her hand over the quilt until she came to a soft blue patch with flowers on it. "This one, Katy," she said, looking up at her sister. Somehow Lucy found the soft blue patch quite often. It was her favorite story.

"Well," Katherine began, "this one is from a party dress that belonged to a girl with beautiful red hair. Her name was Nell, and everyone said that she was the prettiest girl in town . . . "

Before long, Lucy was asleep, but Katherine kept looking at the quilt. Each piece is special, she thought, and she began to tell herself some of the stories held within the patches of the quilt. Memories of home, friends, family and happier times came flowing over her. Mother had been a dressmaker, so nearly every piece was different. Many were fancy silks and brocades from party dresses of the girls in town. Some were from dresses that had belonged to Katherine. One came from baby Lucy's christening gown. One was from a special dress Katherine wore when she was eight. Here a bit of a wedding dress, there a piece from Grandma's apron. This comforting quilt was now the only possession that gave joy and continuity to Katherine's life, and she fell asleep, grateful for its presence in her life and consoled by the comfort it afforded her.

The days moved slowly on, and the little company rolled across the open plains. It was not easy, but they all tried to be as cheerful as possible and to dream of the new and better life ahead. Each night there were the stories from the quilt.

They had been traveling for about three weeks when Lucy fell ill with a fever. Katherine did everything she could to help Lucy feel better. In the day she would sit with Lucy in the wagon as it lumbered along. She would stroke Lucy's hair, smooth her pillow and sing. At night she would tell the quilt stories and hold Lucy as she fell asleep to the sound of the chirping crickets. Katherine's heart was wrenched with fear for her precious little sister. She would draw the quilt tightly around them both, and the tears would flow as she sought solace in the quilt's comforting warmth.

One day late in the afternoon, when they had camped for the day, Katherine left Lucy resting and went to get cool water from a small nearby stream. As she picked up the bucket, a feeling of calm came over her, and she felt that Lucy would be all right very soon.

Katherine walked slowly through the soft grass toward the water. At the stream, she filled her bucket and sat down. The sound of the water was soothing and refreshing as it bubbled over the rocks. Katherine lay back, looked up at the blue sky, and remembered a few comforting words: "This is the day the Lord hath made. Rejoice and be glad in it." *Maybe everything will be all right,* she thought.

Some time passed, and Katherine told herself she had better get back. She rose, picked up the heavy bucket and began her way back to the wagon. As she crested the little knoll and looked toward the wagon, she froze. Three men were digging not far from her wagon. "A grave! Lucy!" she screamed. "Lucy! Lucy! Lucy!" Katherine dropped the heavy bucket and began to run. Tears were streaming down her cheeks, and she felt as if her heart would pound right out of her chest as she finally reached the wagon and climbed in.

She began to shake uncontrollably. The quilt was neatly folded in the place that had been Lucy's bed. Katherine stumbled backward, almost falling out of the wagon. In a daze, she made her way to where her father was sitting near the men. He was holding the now-still body in his arms. His red, swollen eyes looked up at Katherine, and he said simply, "She's at peace now."

Katherine could only nod her head. She turned, numb with grief, and one of the ladies put an arm around her to lead her back to the wagon. "I'm so sorry, Katherine," the older woman said. "We will need something to wrap her in. It doesn't need to be too big."

Katherine nodded as she climbed into the wagon. Somehow she found her scissors. She carefully picked up the quilt, and with a heavy heart, she began to cut it in half.

Ann Seely
Submitted by Laura J. Teamer

Praise to the Women on My Journey

To the women on my journey

Who showed me the ways to go and ways not to go,

Whose strength and compassion held up a torch of light
and beckoned me to follow,

Whose weakness and ignorance darkened the path and
encouraged me to turn another way.

To the women on my journey

Who showed me how to live and how not to live,

Whose grace, success and gratitude lifted me into the
fullness of surrender to God,

Whose bitterness, envy and wasted gifts warned me
away from the emptiness of self-will.

To the women on my journey

Who showed me what I am and what I am not,

Whose love, encouragement and confidence held me
tenderly and nudged me gently,

Whose judgment, disappointment and lack of faith called
   me to deeper levels of commitment and resolve.

To the women on my journey who taught me love by
   means of both darkness and light,

To these women I say *bless you* and *thank you* from the
   depths of my heart, for I have been healed and set free
   through your joy and through your sacrifice.

Rev. Melissa M. Bowers

More Chicken Soup?

Many of the stories and poems you have read in this book were submitted by readers like you who had read earlier *Chicken Soup for the Soul* books. We are planning to publish five or six *Chicken Soup for the Soul* books every year. We invite you to contribute a story to one of these future volumes.

Stories may be up to 1,200 words and must uplift or inspire. You may submit an original piece or something you clip out of a local newspaper, a magazine, a church bulletin or a company newsletter. It could also be your favorite quotation that you've put on your refrigerator door or a personal experience that has touched you deeply.

To obtain a copy of our submission guidelines and a listing of upcoming *Chicken Soup* books, please write, fax or check one of our Web sites.

Chicken Soup for the *(Specify Which Edition)* Soul
P.O. Box 30880 • Santa Barbara, CA 93130
fax: 805-563-2945
To e-mail or visit our Web site:
www.chickensoup.com

You can also visit the *Chicken Soup for the Soul* site on America Online at keyword: chickensoup.

Just send a copy of your stories and other pieces, indicating which edition they are for, to any of the above addresses.

We will be sure that both you and the author are credited for your submission.

For information about speaking engagements, other books, audiotapes, workshops and training programs, please contact any of the authors directly.

Who Is Jack Canfield?

Jack Canfield is one of America's leading experts in the development of human potential and personal effectiveness. He is both a dynamic, entertaining speaker and a highly sought-after trainer. Jack has a wonderful ability to inform and inspire audiences toward increased levels of self-esteem and peak performance.

He is the author and narrator of several bestselling audio- and videocassette programs, including *Self-Esteem and Peak Performance*, *How to Build High Self-Esteem, Self-Esteem in the Classroom* and *Chicken Soup for the Soul—Live*. He is regularly seen on television shows such as *Good Morning America, 20/20* and *NBC Nightly News*. Jack has coauthored numerous books, including the *Chicken Soup for the Soul* series, *Dare to Win* and *The Aladdin Factor* (all with Mark Victor Hansen), *100 Ways to Build Self-Concept in the Classroom* (with Harold C. Wells) and *Heart at Work* (with Jacqueline Miller).

Jack is a regularly featured speaker for professional associations, school districts, government agencies, churches, hospitals, sales organizations and corporations. His clients have included the American Dental Association, the American Management Association, AT&T, Campbell Soup, Clairol, Domino's Pizza, GE, ITT, Hartford Insurance, Johnson & Johnson, the Million Dollar Roundtable, NCR, New England Telephone, Re/Max, Scott Paper, TRW and Virgin Records. Jack is also on the faculty of Income Builders International, a school for entrepreneurs.

Jack conducts an annual eight-day Training of Trainers program in the areas of self-esteem and peak performance. It attracts educators, counselors, parenting trainers, corporate trainers, professional speakers, ministers and others interested in developing their speaking and seminar-leading skills.

For further information about Jack's books, tapes and training programs, or to schedule him for a presentation, please contact:

The Canfield Training Group
P.O. Box 30880 • Santa Barbara, CA 93130
phone: 805-563-2935 • fax: 805-563-2945
To e-mail or visit our Web site: *http://www.chickensoup.com*

Who Is Mark Victor Hansen?

Mark Victor Hansen is a professional speaker who, in the last 20 years, has made over 4,000 presentations to more than 2 million people in 32 countries. His presentations cover sales excellence and strategies; personal empowerment and development; and how to triple your income and double your time off.

Mark has spent a lifetime dedicated to his mission of making a profound and positive difference in people's lives. Throughout his career, he has inspired hundreds of thousands of people to create a more powerful and purposeful future for themselves while stimulating the sale of billions of dollars worth of goods and services.

Mark is a prolific writer and has authored *Future Diary, How to Achieve Total Prosperity* and *The Miracle of Tithing.* He is coauthor of the *Chicken Soup for the Soul* series, *Dare to Win* and *The Aladdin Factor* (all with Jack Canfield) and *The Master Motivator* (with Joe Batten).

Mark has also produced a complete library of personal empowerment audio- and videocassette programs that have enabled his listeners to recognize and use their innate abilities in their business and personal lives. His message has made him a popular television and radio personality, with appearances on ABC, NBC, CBS, HBO, PBS and CNN. He has also appeared on the cover of numerous magazines, including *Success, Entrepreneur* and *Changes.*

Mark is a big man with a heart and spirit to match—an inspiration to all who seek to better themselves.

For further information about Mark write:

P.O. Box 7665
Newport Beach, CA 92658
phone: 949-759-9304 or 800-433-2314
fax: 949-722-6912
Web site: http://www.chickensoup.com

Who Is Jennifer Read Hawthorne?

Jennifer Read Hawthorne is co-founder of The Esteem Group, a company specializing in self-esteem and inspirational programs for women. A professional speaker since 1975, she has spoken to thousands of women around the world about personal growth, self-development and professional success.

She is also owner of Hawthorne Training Services, Inc., a company that develops and delivers business writing and technical writing courses to business, government and educational organizations. Her clients have included AT&T, Delta Air Lines, Hallmark Cards, The American Legion, NutraSweet, Union Pacific, The Norand Corporation, the State of Iowa, Cargill and Clemson University.

Jennifer's involvement with *Chicken Soup for the Soul* began several years ago, when she started working with Jack Canfield and Mark Victor Hansen, giving keynote addresses and seminars based on the *Chicken Soup for the Soul* message. Already specializing in women's programs, she felt it was a natural next step to team up with Jack, Mark and business partner Marci Shimoff to coauthor *Chicken Soup for the Woman's Soul.*

Jennifer is known as a dynamic and insightful speaker, with a great sense of humor and a gift for telling stories. From an early age she developed a deep appreciation for and love of language, cultured by her parents. In fact, she attributes her love of storytelling to the legacy of her late father, Brooks Read, a renowned Master Storyteller whose original Brer Rabbit stories filled her childhood with magic and a sense of the power of words.

She later expanded her awareness of the power of storytelling while traveling extensively throughout the world. As a Peace Corps volunteer teaching English as a foreign language in West Africa, she discovered the universality of stories to teach, move, uplift and connect people. She says she has never felt this connection more deeply than while working on *Chicken Soup for the Woman's Soul.*

Jennifer is a native of Baton Rouge, Louisiana, where she graduated from Louisiana State University in journalism. She lives in Fairfield, Iowa with her husband, Dan, and two stepchildren, Amy and William.

For further information about Jennifer's availability for speaking and training, contact her at:

Jennifer Hawthorne, Inc. (JHI)
1105 South D Street
Fairfield, Iowa 52556
Tel: 515-472-7136 • Fax: 515-469-6908

Who Is Marci Shimoff?

Marci Shimoff is a professional speaker and trainer who has inspired thousands of people around the world with her message of personal and professional growth. Over the last 16 years she has delivered seminars and keynote addresses on self-esteem, stress management, communication skills and peak performance.

As a top-rated trainer for Fortune 500 companies, Marci has worked with such clients as AT&T, General Motors, Sears, Amoco, Western Union and Bristol-Myers Squibb. She has also been a featured speaker for numerous professional organizations, universities and women's associations, where she is known for her lively humor and dynamic delivery.

Marci combines her energetic style with a strong knowledge base. She earned her M.B.A. from UCLA; she also studied for one year in the United States and Europe to earn an advanced certificate as a stress management consultant.

In 1983, Marci coauthored a highly acclaimed study of the 50 top businesswomen in America. Since that time, she has specialized in addressing women's audiences, focusing on helping women discover the extraordinary within themselves. Along with her business partner, Jennifer Hawthorne, she is co-founder of The Esteem Group, a company that specializes in self-esteem and inspirational programs for women.

Since 1989, Marci has studied self-esteem with Jack Canfield and has assisted in his annual Training of Trainers program for professionals. In the last few years, she has been delivering keynote addresses based on the *Chicken Soup for the Soul* message, in association with Jack Canfield and Mark Victor Hansen.

Because of her extensive experience in addressing women's audiences and her background with *Chicken Soup,* Marci has teamed up with Jennifer, Jack and Mark to coauthor *Chicken Soup for the Woman's Soul.*

Of all the projects Marci has worked on in her career, none have been as fulfilling as creating *Chicken Soup for the Woman's Soul.* She is thrilled at the opportunity to help touch the hearts and rekindle the spirits of millions of women throughout the world through the stories in this book.

For further information about Marci's speaking schedule or consulting work, you can reach her at:

The Esteem Group
1105 South D Street
Fairfield, Iowa 52556
Tel: 515-472-9394 • Fax: 515-472-5065

Contributors

Melody Arnett sees everyone as her teacher. Her two daughters and many friends are among her greatest blessings. She works with homeless and second-language students in a classroom that radiates life and learning. As an advocate to victims of domestic violence, she believes in helping them empower themselves. Melody enjoys practicing the arts of storytelling and writing; this is her first national publication. You can contact Melody at PO Box 692, Grass Valley, CA 95945.

Marsha Arons is a freelance writer and speaker. Her areas of interest include women's issues, child-parent relationships, Christian-Jewish relations, and focusing on the positive aspects of life. She is delighted to contribute to the Chicken Soup books including *Chicken Soup for the Woman's Soul*. In addition, Marsha's stories, essays and articles have appeared in *Good Housekeeping, Redbook, Woman's Day, Woman's World* and *Reader's Digest*. She is currently working on a collection of stories about parenting and a novel for young adults. She can be reached for writing and speaking assignments at her e-mail address: ra8737@aol.com. or by calling 847-329-0280.

Sue Augustine is recognized internationally as a speaker people remember. She presents over 100 high-energy keynotes and seminars annually, focusing on change management, stress survival and time effectiveness for professionals, as well as positive risk-taking and confidence building for women. Sue has produced programs on tape and is the author of *With Wings, There Are No Barriers*, the book that tells the rest of her story. She can be reached at Sue Augustine Seminars, P.O. Box 2194, Niagara Falls, NY 14302 or to order products, call 1-888-WINGS-35.

Beverly M. Bartlett, a native of San Francisco, now resides in Cleveland with her husband, after living in Germany for several years. Though she had traveled to and even studied in Europe before living in its hub, her time in Germany was an eye-opening experience. Meeting others, including refugees, and learning their languages and cultures will long be treasured. She owns a customized trading card business. Beverly can be reached at 2215 Overlook Road, Apt. 8, Cleveland, OH 44106, or call 216-791-3726.

Barbara K. Bassett is a freelance writer who is working on several children's books. Her poem, "Angela's Word," is based on a personal experience. She can be reached at 573-443-4343.

Joan Beck writes an opinion page column for *The Chicago Tribune,* which is distributed nationally by the Knight Ridder Tribune News Service. At the *Tribune,* she has been a feature writer, creator and editor of the Tempo section and a member of the editorial board. She has bachelor's and master's degrees from Northwestern University's Medill School of Journalism. She is the author of four books about mental development in early childhood and has won numerous awards for journalism and for service to children. She and her late husband have two children and two grandchildren.

K. Bernard has recently added a master's degree in professional writing to her extensive background in theater and religious studies. She has published a number of articles in local and regional publications, and has written and designed web pages for the Internet. She likes all kinds of writing, but her heart belongs to poetry.

Edgar Bledsoe was born on a farm in northeastern Missouri. He was one of the "Okies" who went to California in the 1930s, when the Depression interrupted his studies at Texas Tech. He had a successful sales career with Kaiser Aluminum Company and is now retired and living with his wife, Marian, in Green Valley, Arizona.

Jean Bole, R.N., B.A., is Restorative/Rehabilitation certified and a CNA Instructor. She is currently adjunct faculty at several colleges, instructing nursing assistants and patient care associates, as well as a Restraint Alternative and Restraint Reduction consultant to long-term care facilities. She is a published freelance writer/poet. You can reach her by writing to PO Box 11, Crete, IL 60417.

Melissa Masters Bowers is a minister, writer and speaker. After seven years in a West Coast ministry, she relocated with her family to the Midwest to pursue her favorite career—being a mom! A columnist for *New Perspectives* magazine, a freelance writer and a guest lecturer, Melissa specializes in topics that promote wholeness and compassion. She can be reached at 511 N. Main St., Lee's Summit, MO 64063, or call 816-246-5799.

Rita Bresnahan has been an educator for the past 40 years, a psychotherapist for over 25 years and a writer for almost 12 months. Her story, "Walking One Another Home" (written while she spent the summer of '95 back in Illinois country in order to enjoy unrushed time with her mother), will be the lead story/title of her upcoming book. Rita offers workshops and presentations on topics dear to her heart: conscious aging, community and the spirituality of the human journey. Rita can be reached at 500 Wall St. #319, Seattle, WA 98121, or call 206-728-5819.

William Canty's cartoons have appeared in many national magazines, including *Saturday Evening Post, Better Homes and Gardens, Woman's World, National Review* and *Medical Economics.* His syndicated feature *All About Town* runs in 40 newspapers.

Fran Capo is a stand-up comic, lecturer and author and is in the *Guinness Book of World Records* as the fastest-talking female. She has appeared on over 76 television shows and 248 radio shows. Fran both entertains and educates her audiences with her high energy and rapidly paced delivery in her lectures, "How to Get Publicity Without a Publicist" and "Humor and Business Speaking." She can be reached at PO Box 580272, Flushing, NY 11358, or call 718-657-8055, or e-mail FranCNY@aol.com.

Dave Carpenter has been a full-time cartoonist and humorous illustrator since 1981. His cartoons have appeared in *The Wall Street Journal, Forbes, Better Homes and Gardens, Good Housekeeping, Woman's World, First, The Saturday Evening Post* and numerous other publications. Dave can be reached at P.O. Box 520, Emmetsburg, IA 50536 or by calling 712-852-3725.

Fr. Brian Cavanaugh, T.O.R., began collecting quotations, anecdotes and stories as a form of journal-writing therapy. Over the years he has compiled more than 40 handwritten journals. Drawing upon this collection, he writes *Apple Seeds*, a monthly quote letter of motivation and inspiration. These journals have also resulted in four books published by Paulist Press: *The Sower's Seeds: One Hundred Inspiring Stories for Preaching, Teaching and Public Speaking; More Sower's Seeds: Second Planting; Fresh Packet of Sower's Seeds: Third Planting* and *Sower's Seeds Aplenty: Fourth Planting.* Fr. Brian is a storytelling motivational/inspirational lecturer. He can be contacted at Franciscan University, Steubenville, OH 43952.

Philip Sutton Chard is a psychotherapist, business trainer and award-winning newspaper columnist for the *Milwaukee Journal Sentinel.* He is the author of *The Healing Earth: Nature's Medicine for the Troubled Soul* (NorthWord Press, 1994), a groundbreaking work in eco-psychology. Philip's storytelling mastery won him two excellence-in-teaching awards at Michigan State University. He can be reached at NEAS, Inc., 20700 Swenson Dr., #200, Waukesha, WI 53186 or by calling 414-547-3986.

Rebecca Christian is a playwright, travel writer, speaker and columnist raised in Dubuque, Iowa. Her work has appeared in over 100 magazines and newspapers. She can be reached at 641 Alta Vista St., Dubuque, IA 52001, or call 319-582-9193.

Dan Clark is the international ambassador of "the art of being alive." He has spoken to over 2 million people in all 50 states, Canada, Europe, Asia and Russia. Dan is an actor, songwriter, recording artist, video producer and award-winning athlete. He is the well-known author of six books, including *Getting High—How to Really Do It, One Minute Messages* and *The Art of Being Alive.* He can be reached at PO Box 8689, Salt Lake City, UT 84108, or call 801-485-5755.

Sharon Nicola Cramer is part grunt soldier, navigator, medic and commanding officer, and she believes that motherhood, not the Army, is the hardest job you'll ever love. She is addressing *Mother Love*, a quarterly newsletter of humor and inspiration, to other mothers on the "senior tour." Her witty presentations to children, adults and those in recovery combine her storytellling talents and life experiences "in the trenches." You can contact her at 221 West Main Street, Cary, IL 60013, or call 847-516-3691.

Lillian K. Darr worked briefly for the author Ben Hecht and for the editor of the *Saturday Review of Literature,* Norman Cousins. She has two girls and two boys and has lived in New York, California, Hawaii and Fairfield, Iowa, where she now resides. She is a faithful practitioner of the Transcendental Meditation program, with incalculable benefits. Five-and-a-half years ago she met the love of her life, Bill Darr.

Mary Ann Detzler is a wife, mother and Unity minister who specializes in teaching meditation, prosperity and self-awareness. She loves to lead women's retreats. As administrator for a spiritual education organization, she often travels internationally, assisting her husband in teaching spiritual healing. She can be reached at Spiritual Response Center, 727 245th PL NE, Redmond, WA 98053, or call 206-868-3643.

Cathy Downs is a reading specialist at East Burke Middle School in Icard, North Carolina. She enjoys each day in the classroom working with students who have reading difficulties. At the beginning of each year she shares her father's story with her students. She can be reached at P.O. Box 1231, Valdese, NC 28690.

Linda Ellerbee is an award-winning television producer, bestselling author and one of the most sought-after speakers in the country. Over the past 25 years, she has earned a reputation as a highly respected and outspoken journalist, while winning all of television's highest honors. Linda's company, Lucky Duck Productions, is rounding out a decade of producing ground-breaking television. Her first bestseller, *And So It Goes,* is recognized as the most candid portrayal of television news ever written. She can be reached c/o LRB Services, Inc., 96 Morton Street, New York, NY 10014, or call 212-463-0029.

Betty Aboussie Ellis specializes in the design, development and presentation of customized training programs. She and her husband/business partner, Peter, devote their efforts to connecting training with the real work people do every day, setting up training for large service centers in the U.S. and Great Britain. Betty is a founding member of The Outsource Alliance. She reports she is in excellent health and can be reached at 8410 Hall, Lenexa, KS 66219, or call 913-541-9267.

Sandy Ezrine is an author, trainer and management consultant. For 20 years she has worked with foundations, universities, federal agencies and private corporations. Sandy specializes in organizational development, employee motivation and problem-solving. She is currently writing a new book, *1001 Ways to Organize Anything.* She can be reached at PO Box 658, Cornville, AZ 86325, or call 520-639-3311.

Dave Farrell is an award-winning investigative journalist and syndicated columnist. During his 20 years as a daily newspaper reporter, he won numerous state and national awards, including the Professional Journalism Society's National Investigative Reporting Award. In 1992, he received the prestigious Mike Wallace Investigative Fellowship at the University of Michigan. His column, *Roadside Attractions Along the Information Highway,* is syndicated by Universal Press Syndicate and appears in more than 30 newspapers in the U.S., Canada and Japan.

Joan Fountain is a powerful and engaging speaker who owns the training and consulting firm Joan Fountain & Associates. A sought-after motivational keynote speaker, Joan has appeared on the nationally syndicated television talk shows of Oprah Winfrey, Phil Donahue, Sally Jesse Rafael and Montel Williams. Look for her inspirational book, *Nothing Bad Happens—Ever*. Joan can be reached at 3104 0 Street, Suite 220, Sacramento, CA 95816, or call 916-454-5412, or e-mail JMFount@aol.com.

Beverly Gemigniani is a certified teacher and a four-time gold medal winner in the Senior Olympics. The Dancin' Grannies have four exercise videos that have been a recommended buy for libraries and by *Consumer Digest*. The D.G.'s have been on *Donahue, The Today Show* and *Arsenio Hall*, and have danced in the Macy's Thanksgiving Day Parade. They also performed at the White House. They dance, entertain and teach unique sitting exercises across the USA. Call 602-895-7052.

Rosemarie Giessinger is a columnist, speaker and psychic counselor who channels past-life information, spiritual lessons, angels and guides for her clients. She can be reached at PO Box 2024, Albany, OR 97321.

Randy Glasbergen's humorous cartoons are featured in more than 25 countries. His cartoon panel, *The Better Half*, is syndicated daily and Sunday by King Features Syndicate to newspapers worldwide. He has created humorous illustrations for Hallmark, IDG Books, NAPA Auto Parts, *Golf Digest, Woman's World*, American Airlines and many, many more. His books include *Getting Started Drawing and Selling Cartoons, How to Be a Successful Cartoonist* and *Attack of the Zit Monster and Other Teenage Terrors*. Randy lives and works in a big old and creaky three-story Victorian house, in a very small town in rural New York State. For more information or samples, please call or fax 607-674-9492.

Diana Golden is a world-class speaker, writer and Olympic gold medalist. She lost her leg to cancer at the age of 12, and went on to take the ski racing world by storm. Winning an Olympic gold medal and 29 golds in World and National championships, Diana became the most successful ski racer in American history *(Skiing Magazine)*. This articulate and humorous Dartmouth College graduate addresses such issues as creating opportunity out of change, weaving strong individuals into a powerful team, and the many faces of courage. Her electrifying presentations inspire audiences worldwide to break through their fears, pursue their dreams and never, never give up.

Elinor Daily Hall is a member of the *Chicken Soup for the Woman's Soul* team. She also is in business with her husband, Ron. Their company, Global Coherence, Inc., markets products that enhance home and office environments by conditioning electricity and electrical devices. She can be reached at 800-871-0078.

Patty Hansen has her priorities straight—being Mom is number one. As the other half of the "Mark/Patty Team," she divides her time between being chief financial officer and troubleshooter at M.V. Hansen & Associates, Inc., and serving as full-time driver, caretaker and homework assistant to their two daughters, Elisabeth and Melanie. She also loves to squeeze in some time to garden, raise chickens and play on the beach. She is coauthor of *Condensed Chicken Soup for the Soul*. She can be reached at 711 W. 17th St. D2, Costa Mesa, CA 92627. Call 714-759-9304 or from outside California, 800-433-2314.

Jean Harper is a pilot with United Airlines. She is married to another United Airlines pilot and is the mother of two children. She is a writer and public speaker whose favorite subjects are aviation, Christianity, interpersonal communication and inspirational/motivational topics. She can be reached at 8529 E. Nichols Ave., Englewood, CO 80112-2734.

Christine Harris-Amos has a history of formal art training. Her art has always had a sense of love, happiness and whimsy to it. She currently restricts her art shows to her home, which also serves as her gallery. Christine met Wally "Famous" Amos on a flight in which she was a flight attendant. They fell in love, and their common love of chocolate chip cookies became legendary. Christine created two cookie dolls named CHIP and COOKIE and travels with Wally and her daughter, Sarah, to promote them. Christine is a very happy mother, homemaker and artist residing on Oahu, watching the palm trees sway in the cool trade winds.

Jacqueline Hickey is a freelance writer living in Rockport, Massachusetts with her husband and three children. She works as an office manager at the beautiful Seaward Inn in Rockport, and is currently working on her first novel. Jacqueline can be contacted a 6½ Rear Parker Street, Rockport, MA 01966.

Barbara Haines Howett's novel of interrelated stories about culture shock in Indonesia, *Ladies of the Borabudur,* is being circulated by her agent. She received her M.A. in Creative Writing from Antioch University, has been adjunct professor at Northampton Community College, and conducts time management workshops geared to the writing life at writers' conferences.

Linda E. Jessup is founder and director of the Parent Encouragement Program, Inc., a family education center in Kensington, Maryland. She has helped to raise seven children, three of whom are adopted. The author speaks widely and has been a guest on radio.

Teri Johnson serves as a United Methodist minister in the Dakotas conference, where she currently co-pastors the First United Methodist Church of Brookings, South Dakota. Teri loves preaching, writing and teaching, and is always looking for tips on how to juggle her 1,100-member "church family" and her seven-member immediate family. She and her husband, Marty, are the parents of five children: Taylor, Alyssa, Alec, Emily and Elliot. She can be reached at 625 5th St., Brookings, SD 57006, or call 605-692-4345.

Carol Kline is a parenting skills instructor. She teaches a course called "Redirecting Children's Behavior" and is a self-esteem facilitator who works with both children and adults. Carol writes articles for local papers and loves to help others write their stories. She can be reached at P.O. Box 1262, Fairfield, IA 52556.

Christy Carter Koski grew up in Weatherford, Texas. She earned her degree from the University of Maryland Asian Division in Misawa, Japan, where she and her husband lived for three years. They currently reside in New Mexico, where she continues to write poems and stories. She considers herself a life explorer, eagerly anticipating each new adventure and all of the puzzling questions along the way. She can be reached by calling 505-356-6967.

Liah Kraft-Kristaine is a philosopher who devotes her life to the subject of human potential. A former practicing attorney and CNN broadcaster, she now speaks worldwide on self-esteem, stress management and soul growth. Author of six books, including *A Course in Becoming* and the bestselling *30 Days to Happiness,* she has appeared on numerous radio and television shows, including *Oprah.* She is the host of a PBS television special, *The Myths of Happiness.* She can be reached at PO Box 1505043, Nashville, TN 37215, or call 800-427-7982.

Lois Krueger is a full-time mother and friend to three boys. She is also a part-time floral designer and is active in bereavement and support for families as a hospice volunteer. She is currently considering working toward a degree in nursing. Lois resides with her husband, George, in Franklin Park, Illinois.

Alison Lambert is a member of the class of 2000 at the University of Pennsylvania in Philadelphia. She is a certified emergency medical technician (EMT) with the Newton Square Volunteer Fire Company No. 1 in Newton Square, Pennsylvania. Ali is also an ocean lifeguard in Long Beach Township, New Jersey.

Page Lambert has written the Pulitzer-nominated book *In Search of Kinship: Modern Pioneering on the Western Landscape* (Fulcrum Publishing 800-992-2908). The book, from which her story is excerpted, is about Page's life with Hondo and the other animals on her small Wyoming ranch. Page's upcoming book *Shifting Stars,* a novel about the West set in 1850s Wyoming, will be available in summer 1997 from Forge Books. Page is available for workshops and speaking engagements, and can be contacted at P.O. Box 5, Sundance, WY 82729 or by calling 307-283-2530.

Jeanne Marie Laskas writes a weekly column, *Uncommon Sense,* for the *Washington Post* magazine. She is the author of *The Balloon Lady and Other People I Know,* a collection of essays. Her work has appeared in dozens of national magazines, including *GQ, Life, Allure, Health, Redbook, Glamour* and *Reader's Digest.* She can be reached via e-mail at jmlaskas@aol.com, or write to 1701 Benedum Trees Building, Pittsburgh, PA 15222.

Suzanne Thomas Lawlor has written hundreds of magazine articles and is the former senior editor of Cameron and Company, publishers of the *Above San Francisco* series. She has taught more than 500 people Transcendental Meditation over the past 24 years and lives with her husband, Tony, a noted architect and author, in Fairfield, Iowa. An avid gardener, she owns a dried floral business specializing in wreaths. Suzanne can be reached at 515-472-3159.

Bobbie Jensen Lippman is a prolific human-interest writer whose work has appeared in national and international publications. She hosts a radio program called "Bobbie's Beat on the Air," which is broadcast locally and in the Midwest. Bobbie is involved with the visually impaired and is also very active in hospice work. She may be reached at 13650 South Coast Hwy., South Beach, OR 97366, or call 541-867-3805.

Diana Loomans is a dynamic speaker and bestselling author who speaks internationally on the topics of self-esteem, communication and the power of laughter and play. She has written eight books including *Full Esteem Ahead: 100 Ways to Build Esteem in Children & Adults, The Laughing Classroom, The Lovables in the Kingdom of Self-Esteem, Positively Mother Goose,* and *Today I Am Lovable.* She is a frequent guest on national radio and television. She can be reached at Global Learning, P.O. Box 1203, Solana Beach, CA 92075 or by calling 619-944-9842 or by faxing 619-942-5260.

Patricia Lorenz is an inspirational/humor writer of books, articles and columns. Her first two books, *Stuff That Matters for Single Parents* and *A Hug a Day for Single Parents* (365 daily devotionals) are published by Servant Publications in Ann Arbor, Michigan. Over 400 of her non-fiction articles have appeared in 70 publications, including *Reader's Digest, Guideposts, Working Mother* and *Single-Parent Family.* You can write to her at 7457 S. Pennsylvania Ave., Oak Creek, WI 53154.

Mary Miller is a marketing communications manager at a Fortune 500 company and the mother of six children. She writes for local publications and frequently delivers speeches to business groups.

Stacey Nasalroad was born in Fresno, California, and grew up in Modesto, California. She presently lives in Zimbabwe, where her husband is running a building company. She helps her husband with the business while enjoying life in a foreign country along with her daughter, Jessica, and her son, Adam. Although living in Africa is a benefit to her and her family in many ways, America will always be her home.

Sheryl Nicholson is an international professional speaker of 14 years. Whether speaking on leadership, sales or balancing our choices in life, Sheryl continues to spice up her workshops with real-life examples like the one in this book. She has authored several books, audiotapes and a computer-based training course for companies on assertive communication. You can reach Sheryl at 1404 Corner Oaks Drive, Brandon, FL 33510, or call 800-245-3735.

Lynn Rogers Petrak is a freelance writer and journalism teacher who lives in La Grange, Illinois, with her husband, Michael. She has written for the *Chicago Tribune, Chicago Magazine* and *Romantic Homes Magazine,* among other publications. Her submission is written in memory of her mother and great friend, Carol Rogers, who died in 1994 after a courageous nine-year fight with breast cancer. Lynn can be reached at 708-354-2854.

Debra Halperin Poneman, president of YES! to Success Seminars, is a celebrated speaker on the subject of success and how to achieve it. Debra's warm yet professional style blends nuts-and-bolts practicality with deep and inspiring spiritual insight, making her a popular guest on radio and TV talk shows and a sought-after speaker for corporations and organizations nationwide. Her seminars have been taught in every major U.S. city and many foreign countries. Debra can be reached at 1520 Forest Ave., Evanston, IL 60201, or by calling 847-491-1823.

Carol Price has been a speaker/motivator throughout Australia, Europe and the United States. She has produced laughter, tears and energy for over 20 years. Her specialties include health care, stress management, real self-esteem, stopping difficult people, assertiveness and making life count. She is published on tape on many of these topics. She can be reached at P.O. Box 8731, Madeira Beach, FL 33738, or call 813-397-9111, or fax 813-397-3661.

Maureen Read was born in England in 1924. Her career includes four and a half years with the British Broadcasting Corporation and a year in Budapest, Hungary, with the United Nations Relief and Rehabilitation Administration. There, she met and married her GI husband and came to the United States. Widowed almost immediately, she later remarried, and she and her husband of 42 years raised three daughters, one of whom coauthored this book! She is an avid tennis player and, at 72, continues to play in USTA and other senior tennis tournaments. She resides in Baton Rouge, Louisiana.

Elaine Reese is a freelance writer in Spring Green, Wisconsin. Most of her articles are reminiscent of families, holidays, the country and the nitty-gritty of everyday life. She can be reached at 608-588-2284.

Lynn Robertson resides in a northwest suburb of Chicago with her husband and two sons. She co-owns an industrial design and contracting business with her husband, Doug, and enjoys interior design.

Jennifer Rosenfeld is currently writing *Building Your Yellow Brick Road: Real Women Create Extraordinary Career Paths*. She would love to hear more inspiring career profiles and can be reached at 212-794-6050.

Gina Barrett Schlesinger is president of Speaker Services, Inc., a professional speakers bureau located in the Philadelphia suburb of Springfield, Pennsylvania. A dynamic speaker herself, Gina gives speeches and seminars on the topics of powerful presentation skills and life leadership time management. She can be reached at Speaker Services, Inc., 491 Baltimore Pike, Springfield, PA 19064, or call 610-544-8899.

Harley L. Schwadron is a former newspaper reporter and public relations writer who lives and works in Ann Arbor, Michigan. He has been a full-time cartoonist since 1985, specializing in business, health and topical cartoons. His freelance cartoons appear in magazines around the world, and his op-ed work can be seen in such papers as *The Washington Post, The Washington Times, The Dayton Daily News, The Los Angeles Times* and *The Des Moines Register*. For many years his work was regularly featured in England's *Punch* magazine.

Ann Winterton Seely is a nationally known professional quiltmaker. She and her sister, Joyce Stewart, teach quiltmaking workshops and have coauthored two books. Ann lives in Taylorsville, Utah, and can be reached at 4890 S. 1575 W., Taylorsville, UT 84123, or call 801-262-1553, or e-mail aaws@aol.com.

Pat Bonney Shepherd is the mother of two. She is the coauthor of the book *Know Your Dreams, Know Yourself* and has recently opened an office supply store/desktop printing service, The Write Stuff, in a thriving East Texas town. She can be reached at PO Box 1173, Pittsburg, TX 75686, or call 903-856-6924, or e-mail TheWriteStuf@earthlink.net.

Louise Shimoff has been happily married to her husband, Marcus, for 53 years and is the mother of three children and grandmother of four. She enjoys golf, volunteer work and world travel. Throughout her life, she has been an avid reader and has passed on her love of language to her children, one of whom is coauthor of *Chicken Soup for the Woman's Soul*. Louise has enjoyed helping her daughter, Marci, with this book.

Andrea (Andy) Skidmore resides in Cleveland, Tennessee. She is a wife of 28 years and the mother of two sons. She has been employed by the Cleveland City School System for 13 years, where she is presently the principal's secretary at Cleveland High School. She has spoken at her church several times on Ladies' Day and writes about the one thing on earth she loves the most, her family.

Charles Slack has been a business reporter and feature writer for the Richmond, Virginia *Times Dispatch* since 1986. He has written articles for *Reader's Digest, Men's Journal* and *Historic Preservation*. A 1983 graduate of Harvard, he lives in Richmond with his wife, Barbara, and daughter, Natalie.

Grazina Smith began her writing career after raising seven children. She has read her works in appearances sponsored by the University of Chicago, the Chicago Public Library and the Feminist Writers Guild. Her work appears in *Prairie Hearts—Women's Writings on the Midwest*, Outrider Press, 1004 East Steger Road, Crete, IL 60417 ($14.95 plus $2.25 shipping).

Doni Tamblyn has written and performed music and comedy for stage and media since 1980. She also travels extensively as a trainer and motivational speaker. As president of HumorWorks, she teaches professionals to use their natural sense of humor productively, appropriately and without fear. She specializes in creativity training and training creatively. She may be reached at 3910 Fulton St., Ste. 8, San Francisco, CA 94118, or call 415-267-3034.

Lynn Towse has never written anything before. She would do anything to mend the hearts of her sisters, Judy and Mary. They are a very close family, and the thought of being published in *Chicken Soup for the Woman's Soul* is very exciting for all of them.

Mary L. Towse is currently the director of corporate diversity for Hallmark Cards, where she has worked for the past 24 years. She has a degree in English literature from the University of Missouri at Kansas City and is currently completing a master's degree in organizational management at St. Mary College in Johnson County, Kansas. She can be reached at P.O. Box 1309, Bonner Springs, KS 66012.

Mark Tucker, a professional photographer and speaker, is co-founder of Awakening Heart Productions and, most recently, founder of Healing Heart Productions. Both of these audio-visual companies have created several highly acclaimed multimedia presentations that have been experienced by more than a half a million people worldwide. Mark and his twin brother, Dean Tucker, have presented their work for countless numbers of spiritual, academic and health care centers throughout the world. Mark is dedicated to sharing his exquisite imagery, life affirming music and touching words to elevate people's love and appreciation for one another. He can be reached at 303 Gunderman Rd., Studio 1, Spencer, NY 14833 or call 607-273-1587.

Phyllis Volkens, an Iowa native, had a unique talent for transcribing life experiences from her heart to the printed page. When asked what she wrote about, she would say, "I write about people and what makes them laugh and cry." Her work appeared in various newspapers and magazines, including *Reader's Digest*. Phyllis passed away on May 3, 1996. She will be deeply missed by many.

Laurie Waldron lives in Arvada, Colorado, and is employed as an executive assistant. This is her first published story. As a busy single mom, she enjoys spending her free time with her three-year-old son. She also enjoys reading, Rollerblading, bicycling and camping.

Marjorie Wallé is a published writer, seminar facilitator and consultant. She manages the Illinois Statewide Radon Program. Under her management, it has been recognized for its public awareness efforts with outstanding achievement and teamwork awards from the U.S. Environmental Protection Agency. You can call Marjorie at 217-786-6398.

Charlotte Ward leads seminars in the PhotoReading Whole Mind System. She trains people to masterfully process the printed page using state-of-the-art strategies described in her book, *Simply Live It Up*. Among them are 40 brief solutions for meeting the challenges of the Information Age. Master practitioner of NLP, certified in using MBTI, and a Toastmaster for seven years, Charlotte speaks and teaches nationally. She is president of Accelerated Learning of Maryland, 7106 Saunders Court, Bethesda, MD 20817. Call 301-365-8112.

Sue West is a publisher, educator, writer and meditation instructor. She has lived on four continents and feels at home just about everywhere. She can be reached at 5540 Fremont St., Oakland, CA 94608.

Dr. Kay Cordell Whitaker is the author of *The Reluctant Shaman* and *Sacred Link* and is an internationally recognized master storyteller/lecturer. In 1974, she began an apprenticeship with two Native American shamans from the Central Eastern Andes, Chea and Domano Hetaka. Her work encompasses corporate, university and private workshops focusing on inner freedom, healing and balance. She can be reached at 4970 Nectar Way, Eugene, OR 97405, or call 541-686-6781. Fax 541-683-6136, or e-mail khww@efn.org.

Donna Wick, founder of The Center for Positive Change in Houston, currently conducts a national seminar series, "Let Your Light Shine!" She has an extensive background in personal development, self-esteem training, motivation and inspiration. Donna believes that no one was created arbitrary to the human race and that we all have meaning and purpose to our lives. For information on her center, write 25231 Grogans Mill Road, Suite 195, The Woodlands, TX 77380, or call 713-364-9824, or fax 713-298-7796.

Sasha Williams is a college student, wife and mother of two girls. This essay was written for a composition course. The topic: something that had a major impact on her life.

Susan B. Wilson is a highly acclaimed speaker whose tailored coaching, speaking and books have inspired thousands to make lasting changes in their lives. Her firm specializes in leadership, team development and improved personal success. Her books include *Goal Setting* and *Your Intelligent Heart.* She can be reached at Executive Strategies, 1105 W. 12th St. S., Newton, IA 50208. Call 515-791-7904 or fax 515-792-1956.

Andy Wyatt has been busy cartooning for more than 25 years. Her work has appeared in many national publications as well as those in countries around the world. She is presently the editorial cartoonist for a newspaper in Destin, Florida, having won several Florida Press Association awards. She studied at Boston University and Art Students League in New York City, completing her bachelor's degree at the University of Miami, Florida.

Permissions *(continued from page ii)*

Phenomenal Woman. From *And Still I Rise* by Maya Angelou. ©1978 by Maya Angelou. Reprinted by permission of Random House, Inc.

The White Gardenia. Reprinted by permission of Marsha Arons. ©1995 Marsha Arons.

Words from the Heart. Reprinted by permission of Bobbie Lippman. ©1995 Bobbie Lippman.

Mama's Soup Pot. Reprinted with permission of *Guideposts* magazine. ©1995 by Guideposts. Carmel, NY 10512.

Just in Time, "Are You God?" and *Who Won?* Reprinted by permission of Dan Clark. ©1996 Dan Clark.

Gifts of the Heart. Reprinted by permission of Sheryl Nicholson. ©1996 Sheryl Nicholson.

The Other Woman. Excerpted from *Woman's Day* magazine. Reprinted by permission of David Farrell. ©1995 David Farrell.

Ramona's Touch. Reprinted by permission of Betty Aboussie Ellis. ©1996 Betty Aboussie Ellis.

The Electric Candlesticks. Reprinted by permission of Marsha Arons. ©1996 Marsha Arons.

More Than a Scholarship. Reprinted by permission of Stephanie Bullock. ©1996 Stephanie Bullock.

It Couldn't Hurt. Reprinted by permission of Sandy Ezrine. ©1996 Sandy Ezrine.

A Goodnight Kiss. Reprinted by permission of Stanley Volkens. ©1982 Phyllis Volkens.

Gifts. Reprinted from *In Search of Kinship, Modern Pioneering on the Western Landscape* by Page Lambert. ©1996 by Page Lambert, published by Fulcrum Publishing, 350 Indiana St., Suite 350, Golden, CO 80401.

1,716 Letters. Reprinted by permission of Louise Shimoff. ©1996 Louise Shimoff.

Martha's Secret Ingredient. Reprinted by permission of *Reminisce* magazine. ©1991.

Be a Queen. Reprinted by permission of Oprah Winfrey. ©1993 Oprah Winfrey.

Home Is Where The Heart Is. Reprinted by permission of Roberta L. Messner.©1996 Roberta L. Messner.

A Tale of Two Cities, And Justice Has Been Served, Taking a Break and *The Wise Woman's Stone.* Reprinted by permission of The Economics Press, Inc.

Excerpted from *The Best of Bits & Pieces*. ©1994 The Economics Press.

Where Do the Mermaids Stand? From *All I Really Need to Know I Learned in Kindergarten* by Robert Fulghum. ©1986, 1988 by Robert Fulghum. Reprinted by permission of Random House, Inc.

The Pirate. Reprinted by permission of Marjorie Wallé. ©1996 Marjorie Wallé.

So . . . What Do You Grow? Reprinted by permission of Philip Chard. ©1994 Philip Chard.

Grandma Ruby. Reprinted by permission of Lynn Robertson. ©1996 Lynn Robertson.

Problem or Solution? Reprinted by permission of Edgar Bledsoe. ©1996 Edgar Bledsoe.

True Beauty. Reprinted by permission of Charlotte Ward. ©1996 Charlotte Ward.

Angela's Word. Reprinted by permission of Barbara K. Bassett. ©1996 Barbara K. Bassett.

Just Say Yes. Reprinted by permission of Fran Capo. ©1996 Fran Capo.

The Gift of Gab. Reprinted by permission of Lynn Rogers Petrak. ©1996 Lynn Rogers Petrak.

I Was a Sixth-Grade Scarecrow. Reprinted by permission of Linda Jessup. ©1996 Linda Jessup.

If There's a Will. Reprinted by permission of Stacey Nasalroad and by the May 1995 *Reader's Digest*. ©1995 Stacey Nasalroad.

We've Come a Long Way. Reprinted by permission of Pat Bonney Shepherd. ©1996 Pat Bonney Shepherd.

No Hair Day. Reprinted by permission of Jennifer Rosenfeld and Alison Lambert. ©1996 Jennifer Rosenfeld and Alison Lambert.

Just Like You. Reprinted by permission of Carol Price. ©1996 Carol Price.

Little Red Wagons. Reprinted by permission of Patricia Lorenz. ©1995 Patricia Lorenz.

My Father's Lessons. Downs, Cathy (October, 1994). *The Reading Teacher*, 48(2), 175. Reprinted with permission of Cathy Downs and the International Reading Association. All rights reserved.

Who to Believe? Reprinted by permission of Brian Cavanaugh, T.O.R. Excerpted from *More Sower's Seeds* by Brian Cavanaugh.

The Marks of Life. Reprinted by permission of Diana Golden. ©1996 Diana Golden.

Soaring Free. Reprinted by permission of Laurie Waldron. ©1996 Laurie Waldron.

Tears of Joy. Reprinted by permission of Joan Fountain. ©1996 Joan Fountain.

Home Forever. Reprinted by permission of Jean Bole. ©1996 Jean Bole.

A Handful of Emeralds. Reprinted by permission of Rebecca Christian. ©1996 Rebecca Christian.

What Women Don't Understand About Guys. From *Dave Barry's Complete Guide to Guys* by Dave Barry. ©1995 by Dave Barry. Reprinted by permission of Random House Inc. and the December, 1995 *Reader's Digest.*

Lost and Found. Reprinted by permission of Elinor Daily Hall. ©1996 Elinor Daily Hall.

Grandpa's Valentine. Reprinted by permission of Elaine Reese. ©1996 Elaine Reese.

A Love Like That. Reprinted by permission of The Putnam Publishing Group from *Move On: Adventures in the Real World* by Linda Ellerbee. ©1991 by Linda Ellerbee.

All the Days of My Life. Reprinted by permission of Jeanne Marie Laskas. ©1996 Jeanne Marie Laskas.

It Will Change Your Life. Reprinted by permission of Word, Inc. Excerpted from *Everyday Miracles* by Dale Hanson Bourke. ©1991 Dale Hanson Bourke. All rights reserved.

As I Watch You Sleep. From the book *Full Esteem Ahead.* ©1994 by Diane Loomans with Julia Loomans. Reprinted by permission of H.J. Kramer. All rights reserved.

Running Away. Reprinted by permission of Lois Krueger. ©1996 Lois Krueger.

Help Wanted—The Ideal Mother. Reprinted by permission of Joan Beck. ©1996 Joan Beck.

Graduation Day. Reprinted by permission of Mary Ann Detzler. ©1996 Mary Ann Detzler.

To Give the Gift of Life. Reprinted by permission of Patty Hansen. ©1996 Patty Hansen.

Mother's Day. Reprinted by permission of Sharon Nicola Cramer. ©1996 Sharon Nicola Cramer.

In a Hurry. Reprinted by permission of Gina Barrett Schlesinger. ©1996 Gina Barrett Schlesinger.

No Small Act of Kindness. Reprinted by permission of Donna Wick. ©1996 Donna Wick.

The Last Jar of Jelly. Reprinted by permission of Andy Skidmore. ©1996 Andy Skidmore.

A Christmas Story. Reprinted by permission of Beverly M. Bartlett. ©1996 Beverly M. Bartlett.

Bush Sneakers. Reprinted by permission of Christine Harris-Amos. ©1996 Christine Harris-Amos.

Feather Light. Reprinted by permission of Melody Arnett. ©1996 Melody Arnett.

365 Days. Reprinted by permission of Rosemarie Giessinger. ©1996 Rosemarie Giessinger.

Spots of a Different Color. Reprinted by permission of Grazina Smith. ©1996 Grazina Smith.

The Wind Beneath Her Wings. Reprinted by permission of Jean Harper. ©1996 Jean Harper.

What Do You Want to Be? Reprinted by permission of Reverend Teri Johnson. ©1996 Reverend Teri Johnson.

Hello, Dolly! Excerpted from *Dolly: My Life and Other Unfinished Business* by Dolly Parton. ©1994 by Dolly Parton. Reprinted by permission of HarperCollins Publishers, Inc.

Finding My Wings. Reprinted by permission of Sue Augustine. ©1996 Sue Augustine.

Grandma Moses and Me and *A Room of One's Own.* Reprinted by permission of Liah Kraft-Kristaine. ©1996 Liah Kraft-Kristaine.

"We're All Here to Learn." Reprinted by permission of Charles Slack and *Reader's Digest.* ©1995 Charles Slack.

Meeting Betty Furness. Reprinted by permission of Barbara Haines Howett. ©1996 Barbara Haines Howett.

Keeping Up with Granny . . . and the "Old Guys." From *Sense and Nonsense* by Teresa Bloomingdale. ©1986 by Teresa Bloomingdale. Used by permission of Doubleday, a division of Bantam Doubleday Dell Publishing Group, Inc.

The Dancin' Grannies. Reprinted by permission of Beverly Gemigniani. ©1996 Beverly Gemigniani.

A Romance of the '90s for Those in Their 70s. Reprinted by permission of Lillian K. Darr. ©1996 Lillian K. Darr.

Bessie. From *Having Our Say: The Delaney Sisters' First 100 Years.* ©1994 by A. Elizabeth and Sarah L. Delaney with Amy Hill Hearth. Reprinted by permission of Kodansha America, Inc.

"Are We Having Fun Yet?" Reprinted by permission of Kim Miller. ©1995 Kim Miller.

Asking for Miracles. From *The Feminine Face of God* by Sherry Ruth Anderson and Patricia Hopkins. ©1992 by Sherry Ruth Anderson and Patricia Hopkins. Used by permission of Bantam Books, a division of Bantam Doubelday Dell Publishing Group, Inc.

Let It Be. Reprinted by permission of K. Lynn Towse and Mary L. Towse. ©1996 K. Lynn Towse and Mary L. Towse.

We Are Not Alone. Reprinted by permission of Mary L. Miller. ©1996 Mary L. Miller.

The Hijacking. Reprinted by permission of author (name withheld). ©1996.

Miracle in Toronto. Reprinted by permission of Sue West. ©1996 Sue West.

War Story. Reprinted by permission of Maureen Read. ©1996 Maureen Read.

Connection. Reprinted by permission of Susan B. Wilson. ©1996 Susan B. Wilson.

Higher Love. Reprinted by permission of Suzanne Thomas Lawlor. ©1996 Suzanne Thomas Lawlor.

I Wonder Why Things Are the Way They Are. Reprinted by permission of Christy Carter Koski. ©1996 Christy Carter Koski.

On Giving Birth. Reprinted by permission of Kay Cordell Whitaker. ©1996 Kay Cordell Whitaker.

A Doll for Great-Grandmother. Reprinted by permission of Jacqueline Hickey. ©1996 Jacqueline Hickey.

Walking One Another Home. Reprinted by permission of Rita Bresnahan. ©1996 Rita Bresnahan.

The Making of a Woman. Reprinted by permission of Doni Tamblyn. ©1996 Doni Tamblyn.

Tribute to Dad. Reprinted by permission of Debra Halperin Poneman. ©1996 Debra Halperin Poneman.

Memories of a Childhood Past. Reprinted by permission of Sasha Williams. ©1995 Sasha Williams.

Threads That Bind. Reprinted by permission of Ann Winterton Seely. ©1992 Ann Winterton Seely.

Praise to the Women on My Journey. Reprinted by permission of Melissa M. Bowers. ©1996 Melissa M. Bowers.

OTHER CHICKEN SOUP FOR THE SOUL® TITLES

Chicken Soup for the Soul

Stories may be *the* most powerful
teaching tool available to us, especially
when the subjects being taught are
love, respect and values. In this book
the authors share a collected wisdom
on love, parenting, heroism, death and
the overcoming of obstacles.

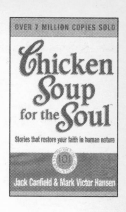

0 09 181956 3   £8.99

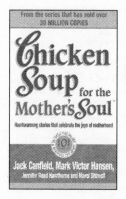

Chicken Soup for the Mother's Soul

Chicken Soup for the Mother's Soul
pays tribute to motherhood – the
vocation that requires the skills of a
master mediator, mentor, cook,
chauffeur and counsellor. These
heartwarming stories celebrate the
defining moments of motherhood –
from birth to letting go as your
children leave the nest.

0 09 181976 8   £8.99

A 2nd Helping of Chicken Soup for the Soul

Another joyful collection of stories full
of shining examples of the best
qualities we all share as human
beings: compassion, grace, forgiveness, hope, courage, dedication,
generosity and faith.

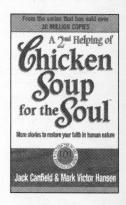

0 09 181966 0   £8.99

Available from all good bookshops
or you can order direct from 01206 256000

OTHER CHICKEN SOUP FOR THE SOUL® TITLES

Chicken Soup for the Pet Lover's Soul

Do you talk to your pets like they're real people? Do you sign your cat's name on greeting cards? Does your dog's wild 'welcome home' make your day? Now there's a book written for you and anyone else who has ever been touched by the love of a pet.

0 09 181946 6   £8.99

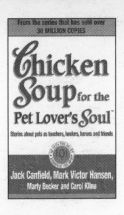

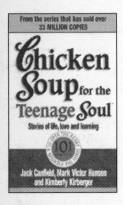

Chicken Soup for the Teenage Soul

Chicken Soup for the Teenage Soul is your handbook for surviving and succeeding during these exciting, but sometimes difficult years. It contains important lessons on the nature of friendship and love, the value of respect for yourself and others, and dealing with tough issues like death, suicide and the loss of love.

0 09 182640 3   £8.99

Chicken Soup for the Soul at Work

Work is an important part of living, whether you wait on customers, run a business or cook for your family. *Chicken Soup for the Soul at Work* is a special collection of inspiring stories that share the daily courage, compassion and creativity that take place in workplaces everywhere.

0 09 182549 0   £8.99

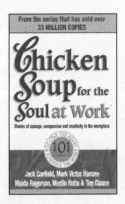

Available from all good bookshops
or you can order direct from 01206 256000

New Title

Chicken Soup for the Couple's Soul   0 09 182548 2